Snored to

A book about how every breath is killing you....

And what you can do to fix it....

Snored to Death

Dr David McIntosh

MBBS PhD FRACS

Adjunct Associate Professor

Otorhinolaryngologist

ENT Specialists

Australia

First edition 2017

ENT Specialists

9/14 Aerodrome Rd, Maroochydore, Queensland 4558

©Dr David McIntosh and ENT Specialists Australia

Disclaimer.

This book and its contents do not constitute medical advice and should not be read or interpreted as being applicable to you or your child's health care needs. In all circumstances related to healthcare, the advice of a qualified and trained health care provider should be sought in all matters. Due to the rapid progress of advances in medical knowledge, the current state of knowledge on this topic may supersede information presented in this publication.

For Adam and Sophie

About the Author

Dr David McIntosh is an adjunct Associate Professor of ENT Surgery in Queensland, Australia. He has a special interest in paediatric ENT, nose and sinus disease, and snoring and sleep apnoea. He is an internationally recognised specialist in the field of the interplay between ENT and dentistry.

He is the founder of one of the largest private ENT services in Australia and runs the largest education service in the world for dentists and doctors on ENT. He also runs the online Facebook pages "ENT for dentists" and "ENT updates for the GP".

With a demand for his services nationwide, he has settled in Queensland's Sunshine Coast region as the place he calls home, as it allows access to his services for people travelling from all over the country (and occasionally from overseas) whilst affording a balanced lifestyle that the beautiful surrounds have to offer.

He holds a PhD, paediatric subspecialty qualifications, and that has been a recipient of a NHMRC scholarship. There are few in ENT surgeons in Australia that have just one of these, let alone all three.

David is also actively involved in providing desperately needed ENT services to indigenous children and is a pro bono consultant advisor on indigenous health to local organisations and government bodies.

When he is not serving the community as a doctor, he is active in the field of physical fitness with a range of interests in various forms of recreational exercise.

Contents

Snored to death

You may have come across the phrase "bored to death" but did you know that in fact it should be "snored to death"? While we are at it "bored to tears" is also something we should be changing to "snored to tears".

Why?

Quite simply, we got snoring all wrong.

It is not cute and it is not good. Snoring is a noise that is made due to blockage of the airway. Having a blocked airway is not a good thing, just like being choked or strangled is not a good thing either. In fact, you should think of snoring as being the equivalent of being choked, but from the inside rather than from the outside.

This choking results in low oxygen levels, which in turn affect your heart and brain. The sleep quality suffers and becomes poor and this leads to being unrefreshed, tired, grumpy, and is often a cause of poor concentration during the day. As a result, people with airway obstruction are actually more likely to be emotional, and have health issues that could lead to an early grave. Even being bored, with reduced concentration, is a symptom of poor sleep quality from snoring. This is why "snored to death" is quite appropriate, in terms of the effect on the heart, and "snored to tears" is representative of the emotional and behavioural changes.

While we relate to the humorous (OK, maybe not so funny for most) stories of wives ready to smother or divorce their husbands due to snoring, there is a serious element to snoring that affects your health in so many ways. What's more it is not just adults but it is children too- to cut to the chase, when it comes to breathing problems at night, it is children more than adults that we are most worried about.

In my professional office, all too often, I am seeing children with a range of ear, nose, and throat problems where the parents have been advised it is OK to leave them be, to just wait for them to outgrow things and snoring is but one example. The problem is that even though a child may stop snoring eventually, there are a range of things that occur within their bodies and brains whilst they are snoring that can leave them with life-long health problems. That is neither a good thing nor a fair thing to that child.

The aim of this book is to encourage parents to understand the whole dynamics of obstructed breathing in children, and understand not only why their child needs help, but to give them the necessary knowledge to demand that help is provided- no more being fobbed off as a paranoid mother or father. This book also talks about adults who snore and why it is more than just a social problem. All the content in this book is scientifically based and references are available upon request.

This book is not only is an educational tool for parents. It is suited for health professionals also, so that we can all focus on getting better sleep and improving our health. Hopefully it is your health professional that recommended this book to you. Either way, read the book, and if anyone you know snores, make sure they read a copy also. Then go see your doctor- if they have not read this book, get them to do it, because until then you will know more than they do- and there is a lot to learned from this book that they should know if they are serious about looking after your health.

Disclaimer: this book is not intended as medical advice and should not be taken as such. It is a general overview on a topic and as such cannot be relied upon as being specific to you or your child's circumstances. All medical diagnoses should be made by a fully trained and qualified health care professional. If you wish to seek a consultation with Dr David McIntosh, you may do so by contacting him via his website www.entspecialists.com.au or the clinic Facebook page "ENT Specialists Australia".

For updates on the scientific research available to the public on this topic, please like and subscribe to the feed from the Facebook page for this book "Snored to Death- the book".

Background

The airway is conveniently divided into the upper airway and lower airway, with the dividing line between the two being the voice box. Essentially it is the nose and throat at the top, versus the windpipe and lungs below. The focus of this book is problems of the upper airway, as it is at this level of the airway that obstruction causes a snoring noise. If the obstruction is lower down in the voice box or windpipe, then the noise is somewhat different in character and is what is referred to as stridor, which there will be a separate short section on, just to be thorough.

The type of airway obstruction this book is focussing on is long term obstruction. So this book is not, for example, about the blocked nose for a couple of days from a cold. It is about blockages that last weeks, to months, to years. Long term blockage is bad for a host of reasons. The type and impact of blockage can vary from one person to the next. Importantly, children who snore need to be managed very differently to adults. This is all explained as the book goes along.

Before proceeding, there are a few important definitions and explanations of terminology. As it is unavoidable that some medical words will creep into the discussion, please bookmark the next page so you can come back to make reference to things, as needs be.

Apnoea- pronounced "app-knee-ah"

This literally means without breath.

Hypopnoea- pronounced "hi-pop-knee-ah"

This refers to a decreased amount of air taken in with breathing. Specifically, it relates to taking in less than half of what would have been a normal breath.

Obstructive sleep apnoea

This describes the situation where there is no air movement with breathing whilst asleep, but the lungs are moving, trying to breathe. In simple terms there is a blockage that does not allow air to get into the lungs.

Central sleep apnoea

This describes the situation where there is no breathing whilst asleep because the lungs are not moving. Basically, the brain, which controls breathing, does not work properly and the usual automatic message it sends to the lungs to breathe in, never happens.

The most politically incorrect but clinically correct statement ever published on this topic is probably this one:

"The stupid lazy child who frequently suffers from headaches at school, breathes through his mouth instead of his nose, snores and is restless at night, and wakes up with a dry mouth in the morning, is well worthy of the solicitous attention of the school medical officer."

British Medical Journal
"On some causes of backwardness and stupidity in children"
Dr. William Hill in 1889

This quote stands the test of time. By the time you have read this book, and absorb everything it has to offer, you will appreciate this quote again with a great amount of insight. The outline of this book is relatively straight forward. In the first section, the causes of airway obstruction will be explained. In the second section, the consequences of obstructed breathing will be discussed. The third section will explain all the possible tests that can be done for people who snore. Lastly, treatment options are explained, with the benefits they deliver elaborated upon.

Throughout this book, the aim is to explain things using simple concepts. As you read through, you will see a great amount of interactions between various topics- these are basically highlighting that there are vicious circles that feed in on each other, making things progressively worse overall. As a result of this, there is some duplication of concepts at times. This is deliberate, as it helps to reinforce the information being conveyed.

Due to the need to repeat and cross-reference back to things, this book is best read with an open mind and deliberate plan. Rather than it being a cover to cover sort of read, it will be better to read, go back and read something again, then progress forwards. By doing so, the interactive dynamics of everything going on will make a lot more sense and be easier to comprehend. So get lots of book marks or sticky labels ready as it will make finding things much easier when you start to cross reference between sections.

Section 1. Normal breathing

Before we can understand abnormal, it is very important to understand normal. It is also important to have a good foundation to build on, as there are so many misleading and confusing messages out there. Whilst the convenience of information being readily accessible on the internet is appealing, the overall quality is so terrible that unless you actually have some science or medical training, you are easily prone to being misinformed. Obviously, this book won't turn you into a doctor, but it will serve as an important reference to have meaningful conversations with doctors, who should read this book also!

Breathing is a natural and basic function of survival. It is so important that it something that is put on automatic pilot. Whilst we can temporarily control our breathing by either holding our breath, or breathing really fast, ultimately the automatic controls take over. Having an automated system is really important, because when we are asleep, we would otherwise stop breathing! (Believe it or not there is actually a medical condition where this happens- the patients need to go on to a breathing machine at night to keep them alive).

In its basic form, when we breathe in, air moves in through our mouth or nose, down into our lungs. While it is OK to take this all for granted, it is my preference that there is an understanding of the science of how this happens, to then make you ready to understand the significance of airway obstruction.

The study of body functions is called physiology, and the science of breathing is called respiratory physiology.

Respiratory physiology involves discussions on the lungs, the heart, blood flow, and 2 chemicals- oxygen and carbon dioxide. There is actually a lot more to it than that, but that's enough to work with for now.

Chest wall movement

For air to get into the lungs, it needs a pump of some sort. To be more precise, it needs suction, as air is drawn into the lungs. And for this to happen, the lungs need to increase in size to form a vacuum effect. This vacuum effect is generated by the movements of the outer chest wall changing the size of the lungs. These chest wall movements come about by the action of muscles, and there are 2 important movements- one is the downward movement of the diaphragm, which sits under the lungs, and the other is the outward movement of the ribs by muscles that attach to them.

These movements make the capacity of the chest cavity larger, which then stretches the lungs open. The diaphragm movement downwards elongates the lungs, and the chest wall movement draws the lungs outwards. As an aside, there are two sets of lungs, divided into a left- and right-hand side.

Stretching the lungs results in little pockets in the lungs (called alveoli by the way) opening up. As this stretching happens, it causes the gas pressure level within these pockets to decrease. The lower pressure within the lungs then results in a lower pressure in the windpipe, throat, nose, and mouth. This decrease in pressure then means that air will want to flow into the lungs to balance things out and make the pressures equal again. As this happens, the airway is usually kept open by a combination of muscles and cartilage.

Sometimes the muscle or cartilage can be too weak, and the decrease in pressure not only draws air in, but can also drag certain soft tissue parts of the airway inwards. The common parts of the airway where this can happen are the outside side walls of the nose, the tonsils (if they are weakly attached to the side walls of the throat), the side walls of the throat themselves, and certain parts of the voice box and windpipe. We will go through these in varying degrees of detail, depending on how important they are to this discussion when we come to discussing airway obstruction.

Gas exchange

When the air moves down into the lungs, it gets to the point where the lining of the lung and the blood flowing through the lungs can almost touch each other. At this point, the oxygen in the air can move into the blood. The use of energy by the body is called metabolism. The body burns up oxygen as part of this process. When oxygen is used by the body, it gets converted into carbon dioxide. This is a waste product, and is removed from the body by transfer from the blood, into the lungs. So when we breathe out, there is less oxygen and more carbon dioxide flowing out than flowed in.

So that is how the 2 main gases are exchanged. But of course, the oxygen needs to get around the body, and the carbon dioxide needs to get to the lungs. This is where the circulatory system comes in to play.

Blood flow

There are 2 sides of the heart, left and right. The left side of the heart receives all the oxygen rich blood from the lungs and pumps it around the whole body. The oxygen from this blood is used up by the cells of the body as part of their metabolic activities. As mentioned above, the end product of this metabolic activity is carbon dioxide. This ends up in the blood which is then transported back to the heart, but this time it goes to the right side of the heart. From here it is then pumped into the lungs to allow the blood to rid itself of the carbon dioxide. In the process of this it also picks up fresh oxygen to then go back into the left side of the heart to do it all again.

In normal circumstances this gas exchange is all controlled and moderated to keep a healthy balance but sometimes a few simple things can start to go wrong and all of a sudden there are issues. So here is a preview as to how breathing through the mouth versus through the nose can be a problem. As part of this we need to talk about a little chemical called nitric oxide.

Nitric oxide

Hopefully an obvious comment to make is that an important requirement for the exchange of oxygen and carbon dioxide is the blood and air must be able to meet each other and interchange their contents. If they do not meet, then the blood can not get rid of the carbon dioxide and also misses out on picking up the oxygen from the air in the lungs. Also, not only is important for the blood and air to meed each other, but it is vital for the amount of blood and air mixing with each other to be balanced. The reason for this is that there is only so much oxygen that a certain volume of blood can collect and likewise there is a limited window of opportunity to get the carbon dioxide out of the blood into the lungs for disposal. If we have a situation, for example, where the blood only goes to the bottom of the lungs, and the air only goes to the top, then there is no mixing, and hence no exchange of oxygen and carbon dioxide.

As silly as the suggestion of blood being at the bottom of the lungs and air at the top may have sounded, there is a graduated amount of blood flow through the lungs, and a graduated amount of air going in to the lungs. Relatively speaking, there is in fact more blood going through the bottom of the lungs, and more air going to the top of the lungs. In other words, there is not a perfect balance of blood and air meeting each other in the lungs. So we need to appreciate the lungs are not an absolutely perfect design in terms of matching things together but collectively they work OK. Part of the reason they work OK is that there are some subtle behind the scenes things going on to adjust for the otherwise imperfect arrangement described just now.

Amongst the mechanisms determining where the blood flows through the lungs to where it is needed most is the ability to control the degree to which the blood vessels open up (and hence moderate the volume of flow through them). Here is where things get to be clever.

There is a chemical messenger called nitric oxide that is made by the nose and sinuses, which comes down into the lungs when we breathe through our nose. The nitric oxide sends a local signal to the blood vessels which causes the blood vessels to dilate open, allowing more blood to then flow through them. Hence, by virtue of the presence of nitric oxide in the lungs where the air has passed in to, there is a message to send more blood towards the parts of the lung where the nitric oxide is present. This is why breathing through the nose is quite important, as breathing through the mouth means there is no nitric oxide, which means there is no signal to send the blood to where it is best to be for gas exchange. It is kind of the body's way of telling the blood to "come over here, where the oxygen is".

Chemoreceptors

Whilst the lungs can do their best to get air in and out, and nitric oxide can help get the blood heading towards where it is needed the most, the lungs themselves have no idea how good a job they are doing. Instead there are parts of the nervous system that are built in to act as monitors for the levels of carbon dioxide and oxygen in the blood. These sensors then inform the brain as to what is going on, and from this information the brain will regulate breathing in terms of the pace of each breath, and the depth of each breath, by controlling the muscles of the diaphragm and chest wall.

These sensors are located within the brain themselves, and in the blood vessels leading to the brain. Each measures something different. And as you are about to find out, oxygen is actually not the most important thing the brain focuses on!

Central sensors

As we breathe without thinking, this is called an automated body activity. It is much the same as how the heart beats by itself. The control system for breathing is in a part of the brain called the respiratory centre. It monitors the amount of carbon dioxide in the blood, and the levels of this are by far the most important thing for it to focus on- oxygen is not its prime concern!

In terms of how the brain responds to carbon dioxide levels, if there is too much building up, this sends a signal to breathe more, to help clear the carbon dioxide out of the body. Likewise, a low carbon dioxide level results in the breathing slowing down, to make sure that effort to breathe is just enough to keep things balanced. In the body, keeping balance is called homeostasis, and the purpose of homeostasis is to make sure that just enough is done to conserve the body's internal environment.

Peripheral sensors

Whilst oxygen is the most important thing to get in when we breathe, the brain actually does not monitor this. The monitors for this are in the big blood vessels going to the brain. This way, if the oxygen levels are dropping, it is detected in the blood before it gets to the brain (all be it by a fraction of a moment, but the brain does not need much time to react to things). This monitoring system is also a safety back up mechanism if the brain sensor for carbon dioxide is not working properly (something that does actually happen in people with upper airway obstruction over time, so it is a good thing that this back up system exists).

Examples of aberrant physiology

Physiology is the study of body systems and how they work. When things are not working properly, we call this pathological. When we understand the process whereby something pathological occurs, we refer to this as the pathophysiology of disease; basically it is the study of how body systems go wrong. We are going to go through all sorts of airway and breathing problems, and their pathophysiology, but to give you a taste of what can go wrong, here are 2 examples that follow on from normal systems that malfunction.

Oxygen sensitivity

As mentioned above, there are sensors in the blood vessels that send messages to the brain about the current oxygen levels. Interestingly, the way the brain picks up and reacts to the signals from these receptors is something that the brain has to learn to some degree. In children with upper airway obstruction, we are worried that the brain may learn that lower oxygen levels are "normal" because that is what it is exposed to at the time of it learning what to expect. The basis of this concern is research done in animals, where newborn rats were exposed to low oxygen levels; as adults their response to low oxygen levels is less than what is should be, when compared to rats not exposed to low oxygen levels early on in their life. In other words, the brain was taught that low oxygen levels were normal and hence was not alerted to a problem as it should have been.

The potential consequence of this is that if we have two adults with upper airway obstruction, and one of these also had airway obstruction with low oxygen levels as a child (and the other adult didn't), then their reaction to low oxygen levels may be less compared to the adult who did not have breathing problems as a child. And remember, low oxygen levels are supposed to trigger the back up system of monitors when the main monitors are not working properly. So this adult is in even more trouble than the one that has a normally functioning oxygen monitoring system, all because the brain learnt early on that low oxygen levels are ok- which of course, is not the case at all!

Right heart strain

As mentioned above (yeah- really- if you've forgotten, then go back and have another read!), the right side of the heart pumps the blood to the lungs. The blood is then directed to flow to where it is most needed by the action of nitric oxide. Nitric oxide works by opening up the blood vessels. In mouth breathing, the nitric oxide made within the nose and sinuses goes to waste. As a result, the blood vessels stay relatively closed. When blood vessels are dilated, the blood pressure drops. If the blood vessels are not dilated then the blood pressure is elevated. With the blood pressure level elevated, it means that the right side of the heart needs to pump harder to move the blood through the lungs.

There is a limit as to how much the heart is able to cope with the increased effort required of it under such circumstances. When it fails to cope, we call this heart failure. We can measure these changes in blood pressure and heart effort. It is very concerning that in children with large adenoids, who are then mouth breathing, we see problems with their heart, even at that very young age. (We are about to talk about adenoids in the next section, so don't worry if you don't know anything about this yet).

Summary:

Normal breathing requires a co-ordination of the brain sensors telling the brain it is time to breathe, and the brain sending messages to the muscles of the chest wall to contract, which leads to the lungs opening up and air moving in. This air contains the vital oxygen for normal body function. Breathing also then allows the removal of carbon dioxide from the system.

For all of this to work, it is important for the air and blood to meet each other and make an exchange of oxygen for carbon dioxide. To help direct the blood to where it is needed, the nose and sinuses make nitric oxide which serves as a messenger to blood vessels to open up, and allow more blood to flow to where the oxygen is.

The best balance of blood to air meeting in the lungs comes about by nasal breathing.

Section 2. The causes of airway obstruction.

It may seem a bit strange to talk about what causes snoring before explaining the consequences of snoring, but like every story, there is method to the madness. Once all the concepts are understood, there is no reason why you can't read this book again, in any order you like- in fact you should read this book more than once, so that the whole picture consolidates. And yes, I did mention I would be repeating myself at times, so this paragraph may seem rather familiar!

Moving forwards, the causes of snoring can be broadly divided into the following categories

1. Something within the airway that is supposed to be there but is either too big or in the wrong place
2. Something collapses inwards and blocks the breathing when someone tries to breathe in
3. The size of the airway is limited in dimensions by virtue of poor facial growth or development
4. There is something within the airway that should not be there, and it is causing blockage
5. There is either poor muscle tone or a problem with the nerves or brain controlling muscle activity, resulting in the airway blocking instead of staying open
6. General health issues impacting on breathing such as asthma and obesity

So let's look at these categories in due course.

Section 2.1 Something within the airway that is supposed to be there but is either too big, or in the wrong place

The airway starts at the nostrils and the lips.

With respect to the nose, from the nostrils there is a nasal cavity on each side that extends straight back to the middle of the head. There are certain structures within the nose that may cause blockage within the nasal cavities. Firstly, there is the middle of the nose internally that separates the nasal cavity into the left and right sides. This is called the nasal septum. It is either straight or crooked. If it is not straight, then it is called a "deviated septum". Having a deviated septum means part of it is going sideways, which is the wrong direction, as it should just go backwards in a straight line. The consequence of this is that a deviated septum narrows the nasal cavity on one side. If it is crooked in both directions, then both nasal cavities are compromised.

The other structure within the nose that is commonly implicated in a blocked nose is a funny sounding thing called a "turbinate". There are usually 3 on each side of the nasal cavity, and they sit at 3 levels, so we call the top one the "superior turbinate", the bottom one the "inferior turbinate" and the one in between is called the "middle turbinate". For the purposes of breathing, the one of interest to us is the bottom one, the inferior turbinate.

The inferior turbinate is a piece of bone covered in soft tissue. This bone comes from the side of the nose, and grows towards the midline. The soft tissue covering of the inferior turbinate goes up and down in size. In fact, it normally goes up on one side, whilst on the other side it is going down, and this alternates like a see-saw going up and down, every 4 hours or so, such that over the course of the day, each side has gone up and down in size a couple of times. This process is called the nasal cycle. We are not really sure why it happens, but it does. When the turbinates are up in size, they would not normally block the nose- if they do, then we say they are enlarged.

An interesting thing that some people notice is that when they lie down at night on their side, the nostril closest to the pillow blocks over, and then they have to roll over, at which point it starts to unblock, and then the other nostril starts to block. This is actually due to the soft tissue covering of the inferior turbinates changing size. What is really interesting is that it is not happening because of gravity, but rather because on the side walls of our rib cage, there are little heat and pressure sensors that detect the position we are lying on, and these feed back to the nose to block it on the side of the body that we are lying on by making the turbinate on the side of the nose that is on the side you are lying on swell up in size. This may help better match airflow to blood flow in the lungs, but to be honest, we are not really sure why this effect occurs.

There are other things that can influence the size of the inferior turbinate, apart from body position. The most common one would be allergies. Specifically, it is a type of allergy we generally call hay fever. The proper medical term is allergic rhinitis. The word rhinitis means "inflamed nose".

Hay fever is pretty easy to explain. In its most basic form, there is something in the air that a person breathes in that the body starts to react to. We call things that trigger an allergy reaction an "allergen". This reaction is mounted by the immune system, which is doing its job by recognising that there is something in the nose that should not be there. The problem with hay fever is that the immune system gets a bit excited and over-reacts. It tries to attack and get rid of the allergen, by using antibodies and immune cells. We call antibodies "immunoglobulins" and abbreviate this to "Ig". There are different types of antibodies, so we categorise them by adding a letter, and sometimes also a number, after the "Ig".

The main type of antibody in allergies is one called "IgE" and the main immune cell is one called a "mast cell". The most important part of the immune system response is that the mast cells release a chemical called histamine (this is why some medications for hay fever are called anti-histamines). When histamine is released, it causes all sorts of body reactions, but the main one related to the turbinates is that it causes blood vessels to open up. In the nose, the rush of blood into the inferior turbinates leads to them swelling up. The other important things about histamine, is that it makes the size of the lower airways in the lungs go smaller, which makes it harder to breathe (this is called asthma). Asthma and allergic rhinitis are linked because of this histamine reaction. Due to this link, it is advised that if someone has asthma, they should be assessed and treated for allergic rhinitis at the same time (and vice versa).

There are other things that can make the turbinates swell. Probably the most interesting is that if you have a deviated septum, the side that the septum is deviated away from, has a bigger inferior turbinate than the side it is deviated towards. Again, we don't quite know why this happens, but is has been suggested that maybe one of the roles of the inferior turbinates is to keep the average airflow the same through both sides of the nose. On this basis, the differences in the size of the turbinates would make sense, as the side that the septum is deviated to is blocked to some degree, and the other side has more room. As a result, to even things out, the turbinate on the side that the septum is deviated towards is made smaller, and the turbinate on the other side gets bigger. The problem with this, of course, is that we end up with blocked nasal passages on both sides, all in the name of equality.

Other causes of turbinate swelling are exposure to cigarette smoke, exposure to irritant chemicals in the air, and something called acid reflux. We will come back to acid reflux later, but for now, just appreciate that our stomach makes juices to dissolve food, and this juice is very high in acid. Sometimes, the stomach juice can come up into the throat, and even into the nose (and amazingly into the middle part of the ear also). When the stomach acid comes up into the oesophagus or throat, we call it "reflux".

So that's the nose, but behind the nose, there is a space. We call this the "post-nasal space" because it is posterior to the nasal cavity. And problems here can cause breathing difficulties. As problems in the post-nasal space can also cause ear problems, we are just going to take a slight detour for the moment and talk a little bit about the ear.

The ear has 3 parts- the ear canal is the outer ear, the part of the ear that looks after balance and transmits sounds to the brain is called the inner ear, and the part of the ear that is behind the ear drum is a space called the middle ear. The middle ear is connected by an internal tube that goes all the way in to the post-nasal space. This tube is called the Eustachian tube. Again, don't worry about this tube too much yet, but it is important as part of the snoring story, so we will be coming back to it.

OK, back to the post-nasal space. The most important thing at the back of the nose, in this space, is something called the adenoids. Now to talk about adenoids, we might as well talk about tonsils, and to talk about those, we are also going to talk about tonsils that most people don't even know exist. But we will walk before we run here. So here is another detour, but it's an important one.

Tonsils and adenoids

The tonsils, as referred to in the general sense of normal discussions, are paired structures that sit on the side walls of the throat, and can be seen by looking in through the mouth. There are also special tonsils that most people have never heard of. These tonsils sit on the back of the tongue, and are called "lingual tonsils". The lingual tonsils are important in the discussion of airway, snoring, and reflux, so there will more about these later. For now, we will focus on the tonsils in the mouth.

But first, we are going back to the adenoids. As mentioned, the adenoids sit on the back wall of the throat, behind the nose. They are in the space referred to above- the post-nasal space. You can't see these looking straight into the mouth. Sometimes you can see them by looking in through the front of the nose (well, OK, you can't, but I can see them because I have the special equipment to allow me to do so), but usually a special torch called a nasal endoscope is needed to get inside the nose and get a good look at them (by the way- I have lots of these in the child size, as the adult sized ones are often too big and uncomfortable).

So what exactly are the tonsils and the adenoids? They are body structures that we refer to as lymphoid tissue. In simple terms, lymphoid tissue has a function related to the immune system. The immune system though, is a massive army of defence to ward off infection. And the tonsils and adenoids are minor players in this game. The role of the tonsils and adenoids in this defence system is most relevant in the first 12 months of life, and even then, they are still minor players. The general immune system is far more important in respect of the immune defences.

Now, you may recall, we talked about immunoglobulins above. The lymphoid tissue related to the throat (and intestinal tract for that matter) is involved in making the IgA type. The most important types for our immunity are IgM and IgG- both of which are made by the blood based immune system cells. This is important to recognise, as not all immunoglobulins are the same.

Now when it comes to surgery, amongst the things some parents and patients have concerns about removing the tonsils and adenoids, is a fear it may affect their defence against illness. The good news is that research has been done on this topic.

So "Does removing the tonsils and/or adenoids result in the immune system being weaker?"

In short the answer is "yes", but (and it is a big BUT, so read the following very carefully), it is not as bad as what some people may try and make it out. Whilst the answer is "yes", it is only a temporary "yes". The reality is that the immune system has a slight period of limited reduction in its capacity for about 3 months after surgical removal of the tonsils and adenoids, but after that, it is back and firing on full cylinders, just as it was before surgery. Furthermore, the research shows that not only does the immune system continue to function just fine without the tonsils or adenoids, those people with sinus infections, middle ear infections, and being prone to colds and flus are better off for having surgery. As an aside, and as will be explained and discussed in more detail later, having airway obstruction actually causes an over-active immune system in some people, so if anything, it helps calm things down once the airway obstruction is relieved.

There is also one other important thing to discuss and it relates to a terrible thing that some alternative health practitioners have been known to say to discourage people and parents from proceeding with surgery to remove the tonsils and adenoids. Believe it or not, they actually tell people that having such surgery increases the chances of developing certain types of cancers. As soon as people hear this fear inducing statement, they are petrified to proceed. The truth, however, is quite the opposite. Not only is there no evidence that surgical removal of the tonsils and adenoids leads to any form of cancer later in life, but the research is suggesting that having upper airway obstruction that is untreated may actually increase the possibility of certain cancers developing. So the truth is completely the opposite to the claims being made. These claims are based on the premise that the immune system serves a function to be on the look out for cancer and to attack it if it develops. This part of the story is actually true, the immune system does do that. But removing the tonsils and adenoids does not diminish that function in any way, shape or form. So, what they are doing here is using a factual statement, and then conflating it with another statement with what seems like a logical next step, but the problem is that it is all made up.

Moving forwards, one thing about the body many people are familiar with, is the old saying "use it or lose it". On that point, you may be surprised to learn that the adenoids normally shrink away and are pretty much gone by the time most people are a teenager. They will sometimes hang around, usually because of infection, cigarette smoke exposure, or reflux. Even though we know the adenoids can shrink away naturally over time, as you will understand from the further content of this book, it is not OK to just wait for this to happen naturally. The main reasons we remove them are for obstruction and infection. We will come back to surgery for tonsils and adenoids later down the track, but for now, this is yet another example of the nonsense of the suggestion that the immune system is weaker or cancer is more likely if you don't have the adenoid tissue- most people don't have adenoids into their adult lives!

In terms of the contribution of the tonsils and adenoids to airway obstruction in children, these 2 elements account for about 80% of all causes of blockage. The question then often asked is "why are they big?" It needs to be understood that size is relative to the total size of the airway to start with. If the airway is small, small tonsils can still be a problem, and if the airway is really large, then large tonsils may not cause a problem. The important thing about size is the space left vacant, as this empty space is the functional part of the airway.

So why are they big? There are lots of theories but the simple facts remain that with any sort of body tissue, there is a natural variation in size from one person to the next- this is why we are different heights, for example. So that is one part of the answer. Another part of the answer relates to limited space to start with, and that is discussed in another separate section about facial growth and development.

So, focussing on the other things that can affect the size of the tonsils and adenoids, the current evidence has investigated the following:

a. infection
b. reflux
c. smoking
d. allergy

Other things such as diet are often thrown into the mix. This is a tricky one as there is no one consistent "diet" from one person to the next. Furthermore, the so called "western diet" that is being made out to be a scourge on our health, has been targeted as a factor in causing the tonsils and adenoids to swell. The problem with this theory is when we go to countries such as Japan, Iran, and Nigeria, their rate of upper airway obstruction is either the same or worse than countries associated with a typical "western diet". So basically, the epidemiology (science of studying disease rates in populations), does not support the assertion that diet is to blame for enlargement of the tonsils or adenoids.

In terms of the causes listed above, reflux and allergy will be discussed later. In terms of smoking though, long story short, please don't smoke around your children. Research has shown that by using special ways of measuring the blood flow in the arm, children exposed to cigarette smoke have altered blood flow compared to those who are not exposed to cigarette smoke. These changes are future risk factors for heart disease. And yes, cigarette smoke contains chemicals that are irritants that cause the nasal turbinates to swell up, and probably cause the adenoids, and maybe the tonsils to increase in size. Smoking around children, by the way, definitely leads to a much higher chance of them having problems with ear infections too. It is not fair to the children to have them starting off on the back foot in terms of their health. Needless to say, it is not good for you either! So look in the eyes of your child if you smoke and decide what future they deserve.

From the above list, as best as we can tell, infection is probably the most relevant factor as to why the tonsils and adenoids get big. But, it is not the typical infection that may first come to mind. Often when people think about infection of the tonsils, they think about raging sore throats, high temperatures, and pus on the back of the throat. This is what we call "acute tonsillitis". The word "acute" in medical terminology means the onset of the symptoms and signs of an illness within the past 2 weeks. But this type of tonsillitis probably has little to do with persistently enlarged tonsils or adenoids.

As you may have then guessed, there is another type of tonsillitis. We call this "chronic tonsillitis". This is a low-grade infection that is pretty insidious, in that it causes a reaction within the body, but not enough to be making people sick, at least not in the conventional way that we think of, as per above with acute tonsillitis. In chronic tonsillitis, there is a low-grade reaction to the infection, with progressive enlargement of the tonsils. Sometimes this chronic infection results in the build up of debris that forms into balls- we call these tonsil stones. They stink like crazy. Some people think it is because they from by bits of food that get stuck in the tonsil and going rotten, but that is actually not the case.

Now to be fair, infection may not be the only factor in play, and we certainly don't fully understand it, but it's the best we have at the moment. In terms of the adenoids, just like we have tonsillitis, we also adenoiditis. There are also adenoid stones that can form sometimes. And the story is pretty much the same in terms of how a chronic low-grade infection can lead to the adenoids becoming enlarged.

Lingual tonsils

The medical name for the tongue is "lingual". The lingual tonsils are those extra set of tonsils lower down in the throat that people have no idea even exists. They are so far down the throat, that you can't even see them looking in the mouth. The best view of them that I get in my clinic is using a telescope that passes through the nose, into the post-nasal space, then down the back of the throat. In fact, this is the way we check most adults for breathing problems. Occasionally we have to do it in children also.

The lingual tonsils can be big because of reflux or infection. The reflux story is quite simple. Basically, stomach contents, and in particular the acid comes up, and causes irritation to the lingual tonsils. They react by swelling up. By swelling up, they narrow the space between the back of the tongue, and the back of the throat. When this narrowing becomes significant, then the airway is compromised, and it affects breathing, especially at night. To make things worse, and we will go through this later in more detail, when the upper airway is blocked, you are more likely to get reflux at night. So, as you may appreciate, there is a vicous circle here, where reflux causes a blockage, then that blockage obstructs the airway, and by obstructing the airway, makes the reflux more of an issue. I have had patients where we have cured them of their snoring and sleep apnoea just by treating their reflux.

In terms of infection affecting the lingual tonsils, it is much the same above with respect to the chronic tonsillitis and chronic adenoiditis. It is all the same sort of tissue, and all susceptible to the same sorts of reactions.

Soft palate

Towards the back of the mouth, there is a piece of soft tissue that goes from one side of the throat to another, with a dangly thing in the middle. The dangly thing is called the uvula, and the soft-tissue is called the soft palate. There is also a hard palate- this is actually the roof of the mouth, and it is really important when we come to talking about the topic of facial growth and development. With regards to the soft palate, this is basically a sheet of muscle. It serves 2 main purposes. The first is to move backwards when we swallow. By doing this, it forms a seal that prevents food and drink going up and into the back of the nose. The other thing is does, relates to the fact that some of the muscles attach to the tube that runs from the back of the nose to the middle ear. You may recall that this is the Eustachian tube. And when we swallow, those muscles temporarily open up the Eustachian tube and allow it to equalise the middle ear space. We will come back to this topic later.

Just as it is there to form a seal when we swallow, it is also there to keep the air passage from the nose down the back of the throat to the lungs open when we breathe. Sometimes, the palate can be too big, and when we sleep, it falls back and blocks the space at the back of the throat. This is an uncommon cause of obstruction to airflow from breathing through the nose. More commonly, the soft palate will shake and vibrate, leading to a noisy amount of snoring. In the past, we used to operate on the soft palate a lot, to stop the snoring noise, often with a laser. What we have learnt now is that due to the many levels of the airway that can become obstructed, we may have settled the snoring down a bit, but made no difference otherwise to fixing the airway, as the site of blockage was actually somewhere else. So whilst managing the palate still has a role, it's not as important as we once thought it needed to be.

Tongue

The tongue is a huge glob of muscle that sits within the mouth and the lower throat. Appearances are somewhat deceptive, as the tongue we can see in the mouth is only about one third of the entire tongue. We call the other two thirds of the tongue the "base of tongue". It is the base of tongue that the lingual tonsils are attached to.

The tongue is a really important part of the body. It serves the purpose of helping us to eat, drink, and speak. Amazingly, it also affects the airway and also possibly affects the way the bones of the face and jaw may grow. So if there is something wrong with the tongue, then there are potential problems with all sorts of other things. The main focus here is airway, but just so you know, if there are problems with swallowing or speech, then the tongue needs to be assessed as part of the deal.

The first thing that can go wrong with the tongue is something that is present from birth, and this is called a tongue tie. The front part of the tongue is attached to the bottom of the mouth. If this attachment is too tight, and it restricts the natural movements of the tongue, we call it a tongue tie. There are all sorts of tongue tie, and it gets very confusing trying to explain them all. The most common and obvious tongue tie is related to a band of tissue in the middle of the under surface of the tongue that is either too short, or attaches to the wrong part of the tongue, but just know there are other types too.

The most obvious time we pick up a tongue tie is when there are early problems for mum and baby with breast feeding. As the tongue can not move properly, the baby has problems latching on and forming a good seal. While not all breast-feeding problems are related to tongue tie, when it is, fixing them is certainly beneficial in a lot of instances. There are all sorts of ways to fix a tongue tie, but they all involve some means of cutting through some soft tissue. It can be a bit traumatic for some parents to watch it happen, but it should not be any worse than the experience of biting accidentally on one's own tongue.

The next stage of life we see tongue ties causing problems is as speech starts to develop. Some sounds are hard to pronounce if the tongue can not reach the top of the mouth, which is what happens if it is stuck down to the bottom of the mouth. There are amazing and instant improvements in speech when tongue ties are released.

The third stage we see problems with tongue tie is the effect they may have on facial bone growth and development. There are 2 bones that get effected here, and we will go through it is more detail later, but for now just appreciate that they may cause the lower jaw to grow out further towards the front than it should, and that the upper jaw possibly grows too narrow. Interestingly, the way the upper jaw can grow when there is a tongue tie is similar to how it seems to grow in some children who are mouth breathers; part of the reason for this is probably because the mouth being open means the tongue does not push up on the hard palate as often or as much as it should. More on all this later.

The other time point we see people with tongue ties is adults. The reasons for this are somewhat intimate, and beyond the need of discussion in this book.

That's everything in the throat that should be there, but for whatever reason one or more of them are either not in the right position, of the correct size, or able to move about properly. So that's the contents. The next section is all about the dynamic movement of structures when we breathe that actually then causes blockage.

Section 2.2 Something collapses inwards and blocks the breathing when someone tries to breathe in

We started this book with an overview on how breathing occurs. Here is a quick summary, just to refresh your memory.

When we breathe in, the muscles related to the chest move. There are 2 important movements- one is the downward movement of the diaphragm, which sits under the lungs, and the other is the outward movement of the ribs by muscles that attach to them. These movements make the capacity of the chest larger, which then stretches the lungs open. By doing this, it opens up the little pockets in the lungs. As this happens first, it causes the pressure level within these pockets to decrease. The lower pressure within the lungs results in a lower air pressure in the windpipe, throat, nose, and mouth. This decrease in pressure then means that air will want to flow into the lungs to balance things out and make the pressures equal again. As this happens, usually the airway is kept open by a combination of muscles and cartilage.

So that is the normal situation. Sometimes, though, the muscles or cartilage can be too weak, and as result the decrease in pressure not only draws air in, but can also drag certain soft tissue parts of the breathing pathway inwards. The common parts of the airway where this can happen are the outer side walls of the nose, the tonsils (if they are weakly attached to the side walls of the throat), the side walls of the throat themselves, and certain parts of the voice box and windpipe. We will go through these in varying degrees of detail, depending on how important they are to this discussion.

Nasal valve collapse

We have already talked about the nasal septum, the usually central internal part of the nose made of bone and cartilage. The septum can be straight or crooked, and we have also talked about the inferior nasal turbinates that change up and down in size. Somewhat surprising for some, the outside of the nose can also be a problem when it comes to breathing. As discussed above, the way air moves into the lungs is because there is an air pressure level decrease in the lungs that is transmitted through the rest of the airway. At the level of the nasal cavity, this pressure is transmitted across the side wall of the nose.

Usually the muscles of the face and the cartilage of the nose work together to keep the nose open. If you want to check this out, look at yourself in the mirror and sniff in. Unless you have nasal valve collapse, the nostrils flare outwards (if yours pinch inwards, then you've got nasal valve collapse- sorry to break it to you). If the cartilage on the side walls of the nose is weak, instead of holding the nose open, it gets sucked inwards, resulting in the nose closing over. We call this part of the nose the nasal valve, and when it falls inwards it is known as nasal valve collapse.

There are several reasons for the cartilage losing its strength, but an important one that leads to it developing is having internal nasal obstruction. When there is blockage within the nose, breathing in is harder. To overcome this additional resistance, people can breathe in more forcefully. By doing this, they generate a higher pressure level, to then move the air through, past the blockage. The problem of this increased effort is there is more pressure put across the side wall of the nose. Slowly over time, this puts a strain on the cartilage, and this leads to stretching and weakening of the nasal cartilage, which eventually gets to the point where the strain is too much, and it starts to then collapse inwards. Think of it like a rubber band that is stretched outwards repeatedly- eventually it loses its elasticity, and does not recoil back to its original resting position.

There are several strategies to dealing with nasal valve collapse, so sit tight as we come to that in due course.

Pedunculated tonsils

Apart from focussing on the size of the tonsils, we also need to look at their position and their attachment to the side wall of the throat. The tonsils themselves sit inside a special pocket on the side wall of the throat. They may be held in tightly, or held on very weakly. If the attachment is minimal, then the tonsils can flap around in the breeze. And this is literally what they do with breathing at night- the muscles on the side wall of the throat are usually relaxed to some degree, so if the attachment to the throat is flimsy, then they fall inwards, and then move around all over the place.

In medical speak, we call a narrow attachment a pedicle, and when the tonsils are poorly attached, we call them pedunculated.

Assessing tonsils for their size, position, and attachment is really important when it comes to deciding on surgery, so there will be a lot more about this in the treatment section.

Lateral wall collapse

Once we move down past the nose, past the mouth, there is a section of the throat that then leads to the voice box and windpipe. This part of the throat is called the pharynx. The boundaries of the pharynx are the spine at the back, the base of the tongue at the front, and then the side walls (which are muscle).

The issues of the tongue base and lingual tonsils at this level, has already been discussed. The back of the pharynx is pretty solid, and apart from occasional bumps of bone growing forwards from the spine (we call these spurs), it usually is not an issue with respect to airway obstruction. In terms of the side walls of the pharynx though, they are mobile and can be involved in obstruction of the airway.

In doctor-speak, things on the sides we call lateral, so the side walls of the pharynx are called the lateral walls. These walls are made of muscle. Usually the muscle maintains a certain degree of activity which keeps the side walls under tension- it's a bit like a drum that is stretched tight to keep it solid. Another analogy is a 6-pack of abdominals versus a beer gut.

For a range of complicated reasons, the tension of the muscle on the side walls of the throat may be less than what it needs to be. When this is the case, the side walls of the throat may get sucked inwards when someone breathes in- sometimes this can happen so much that they actually then touch each other in the middle of the throat. This is called lateral pharyngeal wall collapse. This problem can only be found by using a special telescope that reaches in to the lower part of the throat.

Whilst we are going to talk about treatment of upper airway obstruction in more detail later, now is a nice moment to pause and take a detour from that plan. There are several strategies for managing lateral wall collapse. One of them, like working on those 6-pack abs, is sending the throat to the gym. Now before you get excited, this is not a green light to use your throat more by talking more or eating more. There are studies where patients were given specific throat exercises or activities, and the effect on the airway was assessed down the track. And the amazing thing was that the degree of airway obstruction in adults reduced. To add an Australian flavour to the conversation, one of the methods used was playing the didgeridoo! More later on this topic.

The voice box and wind pipe

Even if the air has been able to get this far through the nose and throat, there is still a chance of obstruction of flow into the lungs. Obstruction at this level does not cause a snoring noise though. Instead it is a different sort of noise that we call stridor. It is important to realise that noisy breathing comes in different forms, as this relates to the different causes. If you go back to the introduction, I made reference to stridor then.

Within the voice box, there are 3 structures that are freely mobile that may cause obstruction. The first thing is the vocal cords themselves. Now these are supposed to move when we breathe and talk, but sometime one or both of them may be paralysed. If this is the case then they tend to sit in the middle of the airway, blocking between 40-98% of the space. This sort of problem is pretty rare, so for the purposes of this book, we won't be worrying about it any more.

The other 2 parts of the voice box that may be an issue are the cartilage at the back of the voice box called the arytenoids, and the cartilage at the front of the voice box called the epiglottis. If this cartilage is able to move more than it should, then in the process of the air coming in, they may be swept up by the air current and fall inwards. This condition is called laryngomalacia. "Laryngo" relates to the voice box, and "malacia" means "softening". Laryngomalacia usually presents at about 6 weeks of age, and in most cases goes away by itself. Sometimes it needs surgery. This type of airway obstruction has little to do with the rest of this conversation, so we won't get too distracted by it further, but I just wanted to make sure you knew about it- you can thank me later.

A final word now on the windpipe and airways to the lungs called the bronchi. These too can be soft and collapse inwards. The windpipe is known as the trachea, so we have tracheomalacia, and the other one is known as bronchomalacia. Again, not really relevant to the rest of the book.

Let's pause to catch our breath (pun intended)

To review our progress, thus far we have been talking about the contents of the airways, and the surrounding structures that make up the airway passages, and how the contents can be too big, or how the passage walls can collapse inwards. Another reason the airway can be compromised is there can be reductions to the size of the airway due to poor bone growth and development. That is what the next section is all about.

Section 2.3 The size of the airway is limited in dimensions by virtue of poor facial growth or development

Think of a room. It has walls, and the space within that room is determined by where the walls are. Within that room, there can be some tables, chairs, and a few boxes. The space to walk around within that room is determined by the position of the walls and how much we fill that room up with things.

This concept of a room is a way of considering the airway. Just like a room, the airway has walls, and the position of those walls is partly determined by the bones of the face. Within the airway space, we have all the things we talked about above, such as tonsils, adenoids, and turbinates. Now if we have a big room, we could have lots of things in it before we run out of space to move around in. Likewise, we can have big tonsils in a big airway that cause no problems. The reverse of this is that we could have a small room (airway), with a small object (tonsils- for example), that does cause limitations that do have an impact.

What's really interesting about the airway though is that it is not a fixed sized room, but rather it is one that grows as the person grows. And as it grows, it can grow to a normal size or a small size, and this is really important- the latter is possibly more likely if there are breathing problems to start with. In other words, if there is a problem with the airway, the way the bones of the skull grow may be adversely altered in such a way that the room does not expand adequately. Essentially, a compromised airway leads to further compromise. Welcome to the fascinating (and very controversial) world of facial growth and development.

When we talk about the growth of the face, we talk about 3 aspects- the skull, the upper and lower jaw, and the teeth. These days lots of people focus on the teeth, which makes sense, because if they don't sit right, their appearance is often not ideal. But it is important to remember that just like the foot bone is connected to the ankle bone (etc), the teeth are attached to the jaws, and the jaws are attached to the rest of the skull. Linking all of this are the muscles of the neck and throat- and if there is a breathing problem, these muscles don't work properly, which then possibly distorts the ways the bones of the jaw and skull can grow. So let's start by talking about the teeth and jaws.

Malocclusion

We have 2 sets of teeth. The first set are called our primary dentition, and the second (adult) set are called our secondary dentition. The teeth sit up inside our gums when we are born, and grow and develop over time. When teeth come out, this process is called eruption.

Just like our hair colour and eye colour, as examples, are programmed in our genes, so too is how our teeth grow. However, just like things like the quality of the food and air we breathe can affect our general health and well-being, there are environmental influences that may determine where our teeth end up sitting. If everything goes well, and the teeth are lined up properly, then we talk about them being in correct alignment. If they are either crooked, not sitting straight, or the top teeth are not coming down properly to meet the bottom teeth, we call this malocclusion.

To put it another way, malocclusion can occur because one or a few teeth are not sitting straight, and sometimes it can be because the top and bottom jaws themselves are not lining up properly. If the jaws do not line up properly, the teeth are not going to touch together properly. And if the jaws are not lined up properly, then the walls of the airway (which in part are attached to the jaw bones) may be wrong also.

Dentists and orthodontists have classified different types of malocclusion, with reference to the position of teeth and jaws.

They classically divide abnormalities of jaw alignment into classes, ranging from 1-3 (or as they prefer to use Roman numerals, I, II, or III). What is really interesting about these classes of malocclusion is that there is an over-representation of various types of malocclusion in the presence of airway obstruction. With nasal obstruction, we see more people with class II patterns, and big tonsils seem to relate to class III. Even restriction of tongue movement (tongue tie) is implicated in the developmental pattern of the jaws. Lastly, it is not just the jaws that are aberrant, even the other bones of the skull may grow differently. All these changes are speculated to be related to the changes in muscle function of the muscles of the face, jaw, throat, and neck. So that is our next port of call- learning some anatomy of head and neck region, and how this all inter-relates to bone development and breathing problems.

Muscle groups

Every muscle of the body has a name. Every muscle of the body has a defined action. The general way muscles work is they are attached to something at each end, and when the muscle pulls, whatever it is attached to, moves. Even though there are individual muscles, they tend to work together, so we are able to put them into groups. The easiest example for this is the tongue, which is actually one big group of 8 different muscles. Likewise we have groups of muscles that open and close the lower jaw, muscles of the lips, muscles of the throat, muscles of the neck, and even the muscles that move the chest wall for breathing.

In scientific research, we can measure the activity of muscles by inserting a small needle probe into them. These needle probes measure the electrical activity in the muscle, which tells us if the muscle is active or resting, and if it is active, just how active it is. Amazingly, there is a difference in the muscle activity of muscles of the face, tongue, and even the neck in those who are able to breathe through their nose with ease, compared to those who have to breathe through their mouth because their nose is so blocked.

What is even more remarkable is that the number of muscles that have an altered degree of activity when the nose is blocked is quite widespread- the tongue, the lips, the face, and the neck muscles all change their level of activity when someone is a mouth breather. It is thought that this alteration in muscle activity may then affect the development of the bones of the face and jaw, and hence the position of the teeth.

To pause for a moment, the fact that muscle activity can effect the development of the bones of the skull is not new knowledge. The best example of this is to have a feel behind your ear, just behind your earlobe. You will feel a lump of bone that sits just behind your lower jaw bone. This is called the mastoid process. There is a muscle that goes from this point, downwards in the front of your neck and towards the midline, to the bones of the chest and collar bone. It is the pull of this muscle that turns the head from side to side. We are not born with a mastoid process. It actually develops over time, as we start to move around our heads as infants. It is the pull of this neck muscle that creates this process. So muscle can actually shape the bones!

Likewise, the muscles of the tongue and neck and face may exert a degree of influence on the bones of the jaws and skull. By understanding how different muscle groups function, we can start to see patterns emerging in the way facial bones grow with reference to different types of breathing patterns.

For starters, let's talk about a malocclusion that fits into a category called Class II (Class 2 for the non-Roman numeral inclined). In this situation, the lower jaw is too short. This pattern is reportedly seen in mouth breathers. Now to explain how this may come about due to breathing through the mouth, it will make more sense if you have done a first aid course (and if you haven't done one, you should- just saying). When you are taught how to do mouth to mouth resuscitation for a child or adult, the first thing you do is tip the head back. This is done to open the airway. Tipping the head back is exactly what mouth breathers also do. There is a commonly adopted posture when mouth breathers sleep, which is to arch their heads backwards. Furthermore, during the day, to compensate for their necks tilting back, they stoop their chests forwards, to keep their eyes positioned towards the front whilst keeping their airway open to breathe through their mouths. With an informed eye, you will start to see this in people as they move about the place.

In this body position, with the head tipped back, it increases the tension within the muscles of the neck and under the lower jaw (try it on yourself – tip your head right back and feel the front of your neck and under your jaw as you do so). This increased muscle tension is transmitted through to the front of the lower jaw, and acts as an anchor, holding the lower jaw back, and hence, over time, possibly hinders its ability to grow forwards. As a result, the upper jaw grows more than the lower jaw, and over time they fail to line up properly.

The other thing that happens in mouth breathers, is that the muscles on the side of the cheeks are put under tension (again, open your mouth and then tip your head back, all the while putting your finger tips on the back half of your cheeks- you feel a subtle increase in the muscle tone of these muscles the further you tip your head backwards). The effect of this is that the cheek muscles pull the middle of the face inwards. The effect of this inward pull is that the middle of the face may then grow narrow. As the skull and face need to keep growing, it will do so by expanding vertically. As a consequence of this, the typical facial profile of a mouth breather is a long and narrow face.

There are other changes that also occur to the upper jaw in mouth breathers. Not only does it get held to be narrow, but there are also changes inside the mouth, specifically, the roof of the mouth, known as the hard palate. The hard palate is mostly formed by the upper jaw bone. In mouth breathers, they commonly develop what is known as a high arched palate. This happens for probably 2 reasons.

The first is that the palate shape is possibly determined by the tongue. Normally, the tongue sits up close to the palate. The muscular action of the tongue is to push on the palate; this has the effect of pushing the palate sideways, or outwards. In mouth breathers, the contact time between the tongue and hard palate is reduced, on account of the fact that opening the mouth results in the tongue coming downward, and hence away from the hard palate. So not only is the palate narrow because of the outside facial muscles pulling it inwards, it is narrow because of the reduced force of action of the tongue to move it outwards. It is a sort of double whammy.

The second factor that results in the high arched palate is that the hard palate is attached in the midline to a structure above it called the nasal septum. We have met this structure already. The nasal septum is also attached to the bottom of the skull (known as the skull base). Amazingly, the skull base may also grow differently when there are airway issues. So again, just like the foot bone is connected to the leg bone, so too the skull bones are attached to the septum, is attached to the hard palate. This attachment to the palate acts as an anchor point, holding the top of the palate upwards. Without the sideways expansion, the palate grows in a shape like the letter "V", all be it an upside-down one.

Another detour now. As mentioned above, the facial muscles all change function when there is mouth breathing. One of the consequences of muscles having to work more than usual is they get bigger. It's just the same as going to the gym. And guess what. The tongue in mouth breathers often gets bigger; expanding into the extra space afforded it. So over time, the tongue (which remember is just a glob of muscle) gets bigger. This is partly because it has to work harder to do its normal job if you are a mouth breather. For example, if you can't breathe through your nose, you quickly adapt to swallowing differently to clear your mouth quickly, and then catch your next breath. The muscles of the tongue respond to this extra effort by increasing in size. Try it for a moment- pinch your nose closed and try and eat and chew a mouthful of food.

OK. Back to the bones.

So that was class 2 malocclusion- a short jaw, a long narrow face, and a high arched palate, and more often seen in mouth breathers. What's really interesting is there are studies of adults with obstructive sleep apnoea, with respect to their facial profile. There is a strong correlation between the chances of having obstructive sleep apnoea as an adult and having a narrow, long face, and a big tongue. In other words, exactly what the mouth breathing children end up with! This yet another reason why finding children with airway problems and treating them early is so important.

The other malocclusion to discuss is class 3 (III). In this situation, it is the lower jaw that is bigger than the upper jaw. In keeping with the concepts outlined above, this may possibly occur due to muscular activity that is not quite as it should be. In this situation the tongue is involved, once again, but in a slightly different way. In children with big tonsils, one of the effects is that, due to their position at the back of the throat, they may put pressure on the tongue, and by doing so, push it forwards. This results in additional contact between the tongue and the front of the lower jaw. The repeated movements of the tongue in this situation encourage the lower jaw to grow forwards. Pretty simple really!

There is another condition that affects the position of the tongue, and this is known as tongue tie. I have spoken about tongue ties already in the context of how it may impact on the upper jaw. The thing about tongue ties is that they are a tricky subject, with some controversies, so it's all explained separately in its own forthcoming section to make it easier to read back on.

Tongue tie

As outlined previously, the tongue is a glob of muscle. It sits on the bottom of the mouth. Its job is to help with speech and swallowing. Its position also may influence both upper and lower jaw development. We noted above that if the tongue is not touching the top of the palate, this may grow narrow, and if it is making too much contact with the lower jaw, this may grow forwards.

Tongue tie is a condition that describes a situation where the mobility of the tongue is compromised. Basically, it is held down to the floor of the mouth. As a result of this it may either not be able to move outwards properly, or upwards properly, or both. It is estimated that 1 out of 20 people have a tongue tie, so they are not rare.

There are different types of tongue tie. By far the most common is where the midline flange of tissue (known as the frenulum), which goes from the bottom of the mouth to the under surface of the tongue, is too short. Another type is where the muscles in the middle of the tongue hold it down too much. This type of tongue tie is hard to diagnose. A last type of tongue tie is where instead of being stuck in the middle, there is a broad based attachment of the tongue to the floor of the mouth, starting in the middle, but then going sideways. This type of tongue tie is probably the most commonly missed sort of variation (and also the hardest to fix).

When the tongue can't move properly, it impairs its function. The more is it impaired, the more it causes problems. The most obvious time point that tongue ties cause problems is at birth, where babies have trouble latching on and engaging in breast feeding. This causes problems not only for the baby, but often also for the mum, as the impaired function causes varying degrees of discomfort to the mum during breast feeding, sometimes resulting in the need to stop. Quick diagnosis and releasing the tongue tie (cutting it) can result in immediate improvements in breast feeding ability by the baby, and delivering comfort to the mum. Other symptoms of tongue tie in babies include colic and reflux. This is probably due to the fact that the poor ability to attach means they take in some air whilst trying to feed. This air ends up in the stomach, and results in the stomach getting bloated. Most mums would be familiar with the need to burp their babies-this is getting the air out of the stomach. Otherwise the air moves its way through the gut, causing distension and discomfort, or the pressure within the stomach grows and the contents come up. The movement of stomach contents from the stomach upwards is called reflux, and we talk more about this later.

The next stage in life that tongue ties may cause problems is in the early years of speech development. The tongue contributes to what is known as articulation. In the English language, it is important for the tongue to be able to reach up behind the upper teeth to produce the "th" sound. Try this yourself- start to say "Thursday" and stop at the "Th" part of it and freeze your tongue and mouth. Pay close attention to where your tongue is- it's touching the back of your top teeth (or at least it should be!). Any child having pronunciation issues should be assessed for tongue tie as part of a clinical work up. Releasing the tie can again have dramatic effects on their speech and people's ability to understand what they are saying.

As an aside, speech problems in children can also be related to nasal obstruction (often due to large adenoids), and also middle ear fluid causing hearing problems- if you can't hear properly, you won't talk properly. As we will explain, those with large adenoids are more likely to have middle ear problems. Also, those with narrow upper jaws tend to have middle ear problems also. In fact, there is a real big overlap between the jaws, breathing, and speech!

The last stage we see children with tongue ties that are causing problems is with the development of the jaws. In tongue ties we see a mixture of changes to both the upper and lower jaw. For the upper jaw, it may be narrow, with a high arched palate, and the lower jaw grows too far forward. This happens due to the position of the tongue and the restriction of its movements.

You may recall that in children that are mouth breathers, they get a narrow face and a high arched palate. Part of the reason for this is that the lower jaw drops down, pulling the facial muscles tense, which holds the jaws inwards. The other reason was that with the lower jaw down, the tongue is away from the upper palate, so the upper palate does not get pushed outwards by the tongue as much as it should. Well, the same applies to tongue tie. In this scenario, the tongue is held down too much, so its ability to push on the upper palate is reduced. So it's a bit like our class 2 malocclusion.

In terms of the lower jaw, with reference to tongue ties, it gets pushed forwards. The reason this happens is that the tongue contracts with swallowing but the force it generates gets transmitted from front to back, rather than up and down. With the tip of the tongue held close to the bottom of the mouth, it hits the inside of the lower jaw. Over time, this muscle force slowly moves the bone forwards. In other words, a similar concept to why class 3 malocclusions may develop with big tonsils.

Adults…
Sometimes people go through to adulthood with a tongue tie. They may have no idea there is a problem, because to them, what they have is quite normal.

It is such a shame that tongue ties are not given the due respect they deserve. These problems are readily identifiable and easily fixed in newborns. The techniques of managing tongue ties are discussed in the surgery section of this book.

Summary

This section was all about how the soft tissues can be dysfunctional. These are normal structures with either reduced strength of abnormal function. An important thing when it comes to blocked airways is there being something within the breathing channel that should not be there in the first place. That is the focus of the next chapter.

Section 2.4 There is something within the airway that should not be there, and it is causing blockage

Polyps

A reasonably common problem these days is sinusitis. Now sinusitis can take on all types of shapes and sizes, and be related to a host of things. One problem we have these days is using words correctly. Patients tend to lump nose and sinus problems together. For example, inflammation of the nose is called rhinitis, and inflammation of the sinuses is called sinusitis. If you have both, we call it rhinosinusitis. Now sometimes it makes sense to lump these conditions together, as the nose and sinuses are adjacent to each other, but it is probably an incorrect approach in some regards. The reason that confusion can arise is that, for example, someone may have hayfever, which if you recall, we call allergic rhinitis. The sinuses may be perfectly fine, and it is just the nose that is affected. Yet patients come in complaining of "sinus". Now it's fair enough- they aren't to know that there is a difference. However, it causes all sorts of confusion with the mixing up of medical terminology with general perceptions of what words mean.

So sticking with the sinuses for the moment, one of the consequences of inflammation of the sinuses is that the lining of the sinuses swells up. If it gets really swollen, then part of it can start to droop. When we this happen, we call the droopy swollen bits "polyps". The word polyp derives from a Greek word that means "grape", and this is exactly what a group of polyps looks like- a bunch of grapes.

When the polyps grow, they may protrude from the sinuses into the nasal airway. In doing so, the nose gets blocked, and people start to snore. It's important to note that polyps usually affect adults rather than children. This is mostly because sinus problems are an issue for adults rather than children. Interestingly, for children that do have sinusitis, by taking out their adenoids, their sinus problems settle down more often than not. Adults aren't quite so lucky, partly (as you may recall) because most adults don't have adenoids to start with (they are usually gone by the teenage years).

The interesting thing about polyps, is they can be associated with asthma (as can sinusitis, and snoring!). So once again, we see this interesting interplay of problems in more than one part of the body.

Tumours

One problem that should never be missed, and this applies to both adults and children, is the presence of something in the airway that should not be there, and is quite nasty- and this is a tumour. Just like big adenoids or big tonsils can block the airway, so too can a tumour. You can get tumours in any part of the airway- the nose, the sinuses, the back of the nose, the mouth, the lower throat, and the voice box. There are all sorts of different symptoms that may arise from such tumours, but one symptom includes new onset of snoring that progressively gets worse over weeks. This is one big reason what people that snore should be assessed by an ENT specialist- it is really important that somebody has a look to see what is going on. Thus far in my career I have seen 3 tumours that presented with snoring that were missed initially because nobody examined the airway of the patient- all they had done was a test called a sleep study. This test will not tell you why you are snoring and certainly won't tell you if you have a tumour.

Section 2.5 There is poor muscle tone, or a problem with the nerves or brain controlling muscle activity

So far we have talked about things around the airway that can go amiss, however, this is not the end of the story. It is important to realise that when it comes to sleep apnoea, there is obstructive sleep apnoea, which we have focussed on thus far, but also central sleep apnoea. The difference between obstructive sleep apnoea, and central sleep apnoea is the effort made to breathe.

In obstructive sleep apnoea, your brain is telling your muscle to move your chest to get your lungs to draw air inwards, but for some reason this effort is hampered by something causing a blockage which impeded air flowing through.

In central sleep apnoea, there is no effort to breathe in the first place. In other words, the brain does not send its normal signal to the muscles around the chest to breathe.

In people with long standing obstructive sleep apnoea, there are gradual and subtle changes in the level of carbon dioxide in the blood. We mentioned this chemical, in the very first section, on respiratory physiology. Feel free to review this again. Basically, the changes in carbon dioxide means that the brain gets used to obstructed breathing over time. So instead of triggering an emergency signal to breathe, the opposite starts to happen, and the brain just doesn't even bother. In people who have both obstructive and central sleep apnoea, we call this mixed sleep apnoea.

Once the brain starts to switch off, things are becoming very serious.

Section 2.6 There is either poor muscle tone or a problem with the nerves or brain controlling muscle activity, resulting in the airway blocking instead of staying open

For everything to work properly as a team, everything has to function properly as an individual entity. For breathing to work properly, the muscles of the chest and throat have to be strong, and the brain and nerves have to be functioning properly. There are medical conditions that affect the brain, nerves, and muscles, and these can impact on breathing. For example, there are conditions that cause low muscle tone. With low muscle tone, the chest does not expand as much, and the throat collapses inwards easier. In isolation these both reduce airflow, so in combination it is a problem that is exponential.

In terms of brain function, again there are conditions where the brain does not work properly. This can be evident in all sorts of ways. For example, the signals to breathe may not register properly. Or the signals from the brain do not travel along the nerves to the muscles properly. With the breakdown in communication, the breathing again suffers. An example of this condition is something called cerebral palsy.

General health issues impacting on breathing such as asthma and obesity

Asthma

Asthma is a disease of the lower airway. Traditionally it has always been looked at in isolation, without reference to what is gong on in the upper airway. It turns out that this may have been a mistake, as there is an interesting relationship between upper and lower airway conditions.

Asthma is known to be an inflammatory disease, which means there are elements of the immune system involved in the disease process. One of the more common elements is a white blood cell called "Mast cells". These cells produce a chemical called histamine. In the lungs, histamine causes the muscles around the breathing tubes to tighten up, which results in the size of the airway getting smaller, which then makes it harder to breathe.

In allergic rhinitis, it is the mast cells that release the histamine also. But in the nose, it causes the blood vessels to dilate, and this causes obstruction to the breathing by virtue of the inferior turbinates swelling up.

When it comes to managing asthma, most medical guidelines in the world emphasise the importance of simultaneously managing nasal allergies. The reason for doing this is that by treating nasal allergies, the patient's immune system is less active, and their asthma control usually then becomes a lot easier.

It is not just allergic rhinitis that is related to asthma. Inflammation of the sinuses (sinusitis) has also been shown to be implicated in asthma severity. Likewise, the research shows that treating sinusitis makes asthma symptoms less.

The most interesting part of the equation on the links between asthma and the upper airway though, is in children with co-existent sleep disordered breathing. When research has been done on these children, some interesting things start to emerge. Firstly, if a child has asthma, it increases the chances they may have sleep disordered breathing. Next, if they have sleep disordered breathing, they have an increased chance of having asthma.

With one problem independently increasing the chance of the other, this all becomes a vicous circle. We think this problem probably comes about due to the common factor being the body generating an inflammatory response. In asthma this is triggered by the mast cells, and in sleep disordered breathing it is a response to hypoxia (low oxygen levels).

So can we break this vicious circle?

The short answer is yes, it seems that we can. Research studies are finding that in children with asthma, once their tonsils and adenoids are removed, their asthma symptoms lessen. It is probably a complicated mixture of reasons as to why this occurs, but the important thing is that we need to look at patients, and not conditions, and assess and appropriately treat all aspects of a patient's condition, rather than have a blinkered view of things.

Obesity

Being overweight is sadly becoming more prevalent. A combination of diet and physical activity determines, in the majority, a person's weight. Do the right things, maintain a health weight. Do the wrong things, and the consequences are a host of chronic ailments. The health impact of obesity is enormous. Not only does it increase the chances of having high blood pressure and diabetes, for example, it also increases the chances of having upper airway obstruction. And having upper airway obstruction affects a range of the body's hormones that encourage weight gain, further adding in to the vicous circle.

Down Syndrome

This condition is correctly known as Trisomy 21. In English, this means that instead of the usual 2 copies of the number 21 chromosome, there are 3. The consequences to breathing are a combination of many of the issues raised thus far.

To start with, there is a tendency to larger tonsils, adenoids, and tongue. This satisfies our first criteria, of something big that is supposed to be there. The next thing is that those with Down Syndrome tend to have an increased chance of part of the airway collapsing in on itself, our second potential cause. Thirdly, in keeping with our classification system of approaching airway compromise, those with Down Syndrome tend to have smaller jaws, and they even tend to have a smaller windpipe to breathe with. It is also not unusual that the muscle tone in those with Trisomy 21 is reduced. Furthermore, there is a tendency to be overweight.

In essence, Trisomy 21 represents the "perfect storm" when it comes to airway issues. It also highlights why there are limitations in what surgery can achieve in fixing problems, as surgery only addresses one aspect of the whole list of contributing factors to airway obstruction.

A note about reflux

Reflux is a medical term that in this context relates to the passage of stomach contents upwards, through the oesophagus (the tube that takes food and drink from the throat, through the chest, into the stomach). The important thing about reflux is that the acid produced by the stomach also comes up at the same time as the food or drink sitting in your stomach at the time. This acid is hydrochloric acid, and it is very strong and damaging outside of the stomach.

People that snore, are more likely to have reflux. In particular, they are more likely to have reflux where the stomach contents come up not just in to the oesophagus, but all the way up into the throat. It can even get into the nose and into the middle ears.

Apart from the damage the stomach acid can do to the throat, it also causes swelling on the back of the tongue, the adenoids, and within the nose. One of the problems with this is that this swelling causes further narrowing of the upper airway, which makes the snoring and potential for apnoea worse, which then makes the reflux worse, makes the swelling worse, narrows the airway more, and so forth.

Section 3. The consequences of snoring

Thus far, we have built up our knowledge on what can cause airway problems. Now we are going to look at the consequences of snoring on children and adults. In doing so, we will be making some reference to certain tests and investigations. These tests are explained in much more detail in the next section, for the purpose of categorising the information on this big topic, so feel free to flick back and forth between this section and the next, especially on your second and subsequent reads (as reading this more than once will mean everything makes much better sense).

To make it easy, we are going to divide the effects of upper airway obstruction up into the body systems that it affects. There is interplay between one system and another, so the categorisation should be seen as blurred lines in the sand rather than well demarcated boundaries. These categories are as follows:

Respiratory
Cardiovascular
Neurological
Gastrointestinal
Endocrine
Immunological
Integumentary (skin)
Musculoskeletal
Urological

Section 3.1 Respiratory

Much has been said of this already, in the breathing section of this book. The most important thing to appreciate is that there is a difference in gas exchange in the lungs, depending on whether you are a mouth breather or a nose breather. In those that have to breathe through their mouths, the blood oxygen level ends up being lower than it should be. This low oxygen level goes on to then have an impact on the cardiovascular system (heart and blood vessels).

Section 3.2 Cardiovascular

The cardiovascular system is made up of the heart and blood vessels. The basics of this system were outlined in the breathing section towards the beginning of this book. However, now seems like a good time to provide a bit more information for those who have a thirst for further knowledge.

The heart is the pump, to move blood around the body, and the blood vessels are the tubes that carry the blood from the heart, through the body, and then back again. The vessels that carry blood away from the heart are called arteries, and the ones that carry blood to the heart are called veins. This is also known collectively as the circulatory system.

The circulatory system is divided in to 2 parts. There is the systemic circulation, which starts with blood being pumped from the left side of the heart, all through out the body, except for the lungs. The veins then bring the blood back to the right side of the heart, and from here the blood is pumped through the lungs, and it then flows in to the left side of the heart. The circulation related to blood flowing through the lungs is called the pulmonary system.

There are some important differences between the pulmonary and systemic circulatory system. The first thing to note is that blood coming from the lungs, to the left side of the heart is rich in oxygen (or at least it should be). From the left side of the heart, the blood gets pumped to all parts of the body, but the places where this blood is pumped to is subject to control (within reason). For example, if you are exercising, more blood goes to your muscles, if you have just had something to eat, more goes to your gut, and if you are engaged in active thought and concentration, it goes to you brain. Now the blood always needs to go everywhere, it is just that there is the capacity to divert it to where it is needed more, when required. There are many mechanisms that control blood flow, and amongst them, there is a regulator that allows increased blood flow to tissue if the local oxygen level drops down. This makes sense, as the only way to boost the oxygen level is to get more blood to flow to the places where the oxygen is running low.

When the blood passes through the tissues, the oxygen is depleted, and the waste products (carbon dioxide in particular) are transported away from the tissues, back to the right side of the heart. From the right side of the heart, all the blood needs to pass through the lungs. This makes sense, as the blood needs to pick up fresh oxygen, and at the same time dump the carbon dioxide off.

It will make sense as I explain it slowly, but if the oxygen level in part of the lung is low, then the blood is diverted away from that part of the lung. This is quite different to the systemic circulation, and this is because there is a difference of intentions of the two circulatory systems. In the systemic circulation, we want the blood going to where the oxygen is low, to replenish things, whereas in the lungs, we want to collect as much new oxygen as we can.

The changes in the size of blood vessels determine the rate of blood flow. Make the blood vessels wider, and more blood passes, make then narrower, and less blood passes. This is OK for the systemic circulation because there are plenty of places for the blood to be spread around. It is potentially somewhat more problematic for the pulmonary system though. In the circumstance of low oxygen in the lungs that is widespread, rather than localised (such as in mouth breathing), then rather than some of the blood vessels narrowing down, all of the blood vessels are narrow.

As the blood has no other place to go, the right side of the heart has to force the blood through these narrow vessels. To do that it needs to pump harder. By pumping harder, the pressure of the blood in the pulmonary system increases. We call high blood pressure hypertension, and in the pulmonary system the correct term is pulmonary hypertension. The heart has the ability to cope with only so much, and the effort required to get the blood through the blood vessels becomes too much, then the heart starts to fail. This is called right heart failure, or "cor pulmonale".

So that is the pulmonary system and right side of the heart malfunctioning. Now what about the systemic circulation and the left side of the heart? Well it turns out we have problems there too.

When we talk about the systemic circulation, it is important to understand that the blood vessels can change their size, to help divert blood to where it needs to be. For example, if you have just eaten, then blood will be directed to your gut to help pick up the nutrients being processed from what you have had to eat. The changes in the size of the blood vessels are brought about by the contraction and relaxation of little muscles around the blood vessels. This is called endothelial muscle. Normally this muscle behaves in a very rigid and orderly way. But in children that snore, is doesn't function properly- we call this endothelial dysfunction. The result of this is that the control of blood flow through the body becomes inappropriate. This slowly leads to the walls of the arteries getting harder, and stiffer, this then leads to high blood pressure.

The other thing that happens is that the body goes into a semi-permanent state of panic due to the lower oxygen levels. This panic results in the release of stress hormones from a gland near the kidney called the adrenal gland. One of these chemicals released is called adrenaline. Adrenaline makes the heart pump harder and faster, and also causes the endothelial muscles to contract. These changes all put the blood pressure up too. There is more about adrenaline in the section on the endocrine system (the endocrine system is all about hormones).

In adults with high blood pressure we try and find a cause of the elevation. When we do, we call this secondary hypertension, meaning the high blood pressure is following on from an identifiable cause. When we can't find a cause, we call this primary hypertension. Primary hypertension is by far the most common type of high blood pressure in adults. Interestingly, we have growing evidence that having had sleep disordered breathing as a child leads to having primary hypertension as an adult. The thing that is super important about all of this is that the research shows that if you intervene early in children, and fix their upper airway obstruction, then the endothelial dysfunction and systemic high blood pressure all sorts itself out and goes away. This is yet another reason for not leaving children to sort themselves out over time.

Another problem that can go wrong with the heart is that the control system ensuring regular heart rhythms can short circuit. When the heart beat is out of rhythm, we call this an arrhythmia. In adults presenting with a certain type of arrhythmia called atrial fibrillation, it is now recommended that they be screed for sleep apnoea. There are other types of arrhythmias associated with sleep apnoea, but this is by far the most common.

Section 3.3 Neurological

This is everything to do with the brain. There is a little bit of overlap with the muscular system, but I will try and keep these separate as best I can, for the sake of categorising things.

When it comes to the brain and neurological system, there is the brain, the motor nerves, the sensory nerves, the autonomic nerves.

Motor

The motor system consists of the brain, that sends nerves to the muscles, which then twitch, and those twitches are what we call movement. The most delicate of movements we call fine motor skills. The ability to perform fine movements is related to constant feedback between the muscles, joints, and skin sensors to the spine and brain. This co-ordination is something the brain learns and adapts to over time. But of course if it learns the wrong things early, these dysfunctions can persist.

When we talked about points of airway obstruction, we mentioned the muscles around the throat. A study in rats, where they deliberately intermittently reduced the amount of oxygen they were getting, resulted in muscles around the throat to become weaker. Even when they then topped up the oxygen levels back to normal, this muscle weakness persisted. Part of the reason for this is that it is not just the muscle that is damaged, but even the nerves to these muscles may be sustaining damage due to the hypoxia and maybe even just by the vibration effect of snoring.

Sensory

When we talk about the senses, we talk about the general senses and the special senses. In the context of sleep, the senses to be talked about are the general sense of touch, and the specific special senses of smell, hearing, and sight. So let's start with general touch first.

Most people know about the sense of touch. It helps us feel things. It's typical to think about this sense in the context of the skin. But we also have this in our throats- and what is really interesting is when this is tested, the sense of touch on the back of the palate is reduced in those who have lower oxygen levels at night. Furthermore, the more the oxygen level goes down, the more sense of touch you also lose too.

Sense of smell

To be able to smell something, the nose must be clear, the nerve endings that come from the brain into the nose must be working properly, and the brain itself must then work properly too. So the first, obvious thing that can go wrong is that the nose is blocked-this is something we have gone over already when we talked about the septum and turbinates and sinuses.

To make the conversation more interesting though, is that it is not just odours passing from the front of the nostrils into the nasal cavity that can be detected, but ones in the throat can come up through the back of the nose, and also be detected. In adults with sleep apnoea, the research has shown that the worse the sleep apnoea score, the worse the sense of smell is. And like the old saying of use it or lose it, this seems to relate somehow to the reduction in size of the nerves that are there to detect the sense of smell. It is possible that these nerves are shrinking down in size.

To round off this part of the conversation, studies have shown that having big tonsils reduces the ability to detect odours via the back of the nose. So if there are big tonsils plus some form of nasal obstruction otherwise, then the sense of smell suffers in both regards. In children, there is a measured improvement in the sense of smell once their tonsils and adenoids are removed. These changes in the sense of smell may also relate to observed changes in children diets once they have surgery. Rather than relying on the basic sense of taste, they have a better appreciation of the flavours of food.

Hearing

The sense of hearing involves picking up the air pressure waves in the environment, and it then being sent to the brain, where it is translated into what we comprehend as sound.

In children with upper airway obstruction, there is an over-representation in the incidence of middle ear problems. The most relevant middle ear problem is the accumulation of fluid in the middle ear space. This then compromises the hearing, by reducing the amount of sound transmitted from the ear drum to the inner ear.

Middle ear fluid will build up and persist if there is a problem with the Eustachian tube. This is the tube that runs to the back of the nose. We used to think that it was large adenoids in the post-nasal space that compromised Eustachian tube function, but we know better understand that it is the abnormal growth of the facial bones and palate that impacts on the ability of the Eustachian tube to work properly.

Auditory processing

In auditory processing disorders, there is not a problem in the picking up of sound, but rather the translation of it. The most common reason (we think) that children develop an auditory processing problem is a lack of brain stimulation by sound in the early years of life due to a build up of middle ear fluid. As mentioned earlier, this does occur in children with upper airway obstruction rather more frequently than in children who do not have airway problems. Furthermore, there are probably central brain changes that are caused by the intermittent hypoxia that affects the brain development, so we are left with children who can hear quite well, but do not understand what they are hearing. Auditory processing disorders do not show up on normal hearing tests. The children need to have a special test, but the problem is we can't test them until they are about 7 years old with the standard tests that we currently utilise.

There is special testing that we can do at an earlier age for auditory processing problems, but this is more for research at the moment than for clinical use. In an important study of children that were habitual snorers, they found that the way the brain processed sounds was abnormal. So again, even mild elements of sleep disordered breathing are having an impact upon the brain's ability to function during the day.

Visual

It is said that the eyes are the window to the soul. They are also a window through which we can look and see what is going on in the brain. The reason for this is that the nerve that carries the messages from our eye to our brain can be visualised by looking through the pupil of the eye itself. We can take pictures of the nerve, measure the size of the nerve, and all sorts of other cool things. We call this part of the back of the eye the optic disc.

Using a special bit of technology called optical coherence tomography, we can measure the size of the nerve fibres (called the retinal nerve fibre layer). In a study of adults with sleep apnoea, it was found that if they had severe obstruction, their nerve fibre layer was decreased. They also tested these patient's visual fields. The visual field is basically how much of what is in front of your eyes that you can see. And in all patients with sleep apnoea, the size of their visual fields was decreased. This all suggests that the nerve fibres are dying off, or degenerating. This is not a good thing, to say the least. And another study that monitored adults with OSA found that 12 months down the track, the degeneration had progressed to be more evident than it had first been. Sadly once this damage is done, it is irreversible.

When I wrote the first draft of this book the research indicated that airway problems in children did not result in the changes to the eye described above. Unfortunately the more recent research has shown children do in fact have damage to the nerve fibres to the eye, and this is permanent. So it again emphasises the importance of early intervention and the flaw in suggesting they will outgrow airway obstruction.

Sleep apnoea has also been suggested to be related to the development of an eye condition called glaucoma. This is a condition where the fluid pressure level within the eyeball itself can get too high. Glaucoma is known to cause permanent nerve damage to the nerves of vision. It is thought this occurs due to the hypoxic damage to the nerves plus the increased pressure in the eyeball reducing the blood supply to the nerve. So again, airway obstruction is not a good thing to have, and not a good thing to leave to chance.

There are other problems related to the eye that are associated with OSA in adults. The first of these is something called floppy eyelid syndrome. This is where the eyelids become so stretched that they can actually flip up over on top of themselves. It tends to affect the eye that is on the same side that the patient favours sleeping on, and with the eyelid lifted open, they have get a dry irritated eye.

A more serious condition is something called central serous chorioretinopathy. In English, this is a sudden accumulation of fluid under the sensory cells in the back of the eyeball. This results in mild-moderate vision impairment, and whilst it can get better, it may take 4 months to do so, and it is possible that by treating sleep apnoea, the vision may improve faster than it would otherwise.

A more significant condition is something called non-arteritic anterior ischaemic optic neuropathy. Quite a mouthful. Easily explained. Think of it as being like a stroke of the nerves of vision. It often presents with people waking up one morning with half of their vision gone. And there is no known cure for this condition. Not really worth taking a chance on this is it?

It is now part of the recommendations of eye specialists that any adults diagnosed with obstructive sleep apnoea should be sent for an eye specialist assessment to look for these sorts of problems, before it is too late. The above should make it clear as to why doing so is a very good idea.

Autonomic system

There is part of the nervous system that basically does its own thing, and we can't really control it. This is called the autonomic nervous system. It is divided up into a sympathetic system (excited, active system) and the parasympathetic system (tends to be calm and relaxed). What is interesting is that in studies where either the oxygen levels are decreased or the carbon dioxide levels increased, the sympathetic system is activated. Furthermore, this is more evident if the lungs are not expanding properly, compared to taking in full, deep breaths. So not only is important to get a good breath in, to fill the lungs, but it is important that the air is delivered via the nose.

The activation of the sympathetic system results in the stimulation of the small muscles around the arteries in the systemic circulation. This leads to high blood pressure.

As we have gone through much of this already, I won't repeat myself further.

Memory

There are certain parts of the brain that deal with short term memory, and parts that deal with long term memory. To get to long term memory, it needs to go through short term memory processing first. These days we can measure brain activity using special scans. We have done this in both children and adults who have upper airway obstruction. In the studies done, it shows that the parts of the brain that relate to memory are not working properly. In fact in several popular books written for the public about how to improve your brain function, they often emphasize the importance of good quality sleep and making sure you have been checked over for sleep apnoea if you are starting to notice brain fog or so called senior moments creep in to your day.

Likewise, we can measure the parts of the brain that regulate our behaviour and maintain concentration, and again, these are not working properly. In children we sometimes see their behaviour as being so erratic that they are given a diagnosis of Attention Deficit Disorder (also known as Attention Deficit Hyperactive Disorder). It is now estimated that at least 25% and maybe as much as 50% of children with ADHD actually have sleep disordered breathing. There are a multitude of studies showing that children treated for airway obstruction have their so called ADHD go away over a few months. It is so important that children are given the correct diagnosis and the cause is managed, not the symptoms.

Section 3.4 Gastrointestinal

Reflux

The gastrointestinal tract technically starts at the mouth and goes all the way to the rear end. One condition we have touched on already is reflux. This is the condition whereby the contents of the stomach pass upwards, back into the oesophagus. People with sleep disordered breathing have increased chance of reflux, and having reflux increases your chances of sleep disordered breathing.

I spoke about reflux when we discussed the lingual tonsils. I also mentioned reflux when it comes to middle ear problems. Reflux is a commonly missed problem, sometimes because the symptoms are rather subtle. There is more than enough mentioned about reflux already that does not need repeating.

Gut bacteria

There has been an emerging understanding that the bacteria that live in our intestines affect our bodies. Thus far we are finding relationships with mood, cognition, and obesity. It also seems to relate to behaviour, such as eating behaviour, mood, and sleep. It remains to be seen how sleep may inter-relate with this, but there is an animal study showing that when rats are deprived of sleep, there is a shift in the production of certain chemicals, possibly by the gut bacteria, that are harmful to health. There is also one study in children that looked at a particular inflammatory group of chemicals called lipopolysaccharides. In children with sleep apnoea, this was increased, and it was suggested that these chemicals may be coming from the gut bacteria.

There is evidence that sleep disordered breathing can affect the gut bacteria. In a mouse study, the mice were exposed to intermittent hypoxia. There was a significant effect on the gut bacteria in these mice, with changes in the numbers of and proportions of bacteria present. Now to be technical for a moment, bacteria known as Firmicutes went up, and Bacteriodetes and Proteobacteria went down. Here is where it gets even more interesting- a study in rats has shown that having a high Firmicutes to Bacteriodiotes ratio can increase the blood pressure, and when they used an antibiotic to rebalance the gut bacteria ratio, the blood pressure went down to normal. Incredible stuff!

As a last point of interest, babies that succumb to sudden infant death syndrome also have altered gut bacteria when compared to babies who are alive and well.

This area is so very interesting and may well be an important missing piece of the puzzle in why environmental factors affect our health. It may possibly be via the actions of these gut bacteria. The fact that these bacteria may even be able to exert some form of mind control over us is quite astounding too. One day I hope to write a book purely on gut bacteria and health. It should make for an interesting perspective to the way we view our health and wellbeing.

Section 3.5 Endocrine and metabolic system

The body produces hormones- this is called the endocrine system. The body also processes food into nutrients and uses these for energy. This is called the metabolic system. And both of these go haywire in those with sleep disordered breathing. Let's go through some of these to give you an idea on the breadth of the problem.

Iron

Iron is an element that is very important in the manufacturing of the red blood cells. These are the cells that carry oxygen around the body. If you do not have enough iron, you may not make enough red blood cells, and if this happens, then you can't carry enough oxygen around. A low red blood cell count is called anaemia, and if it is caused by low iron, it is called iron deficiency anaemia. Given that low oxygen levels is a consequence of sleep disordered breathing, it would not be good if low iron was thrown in to the mix. Unfortunately, that is exactly what happens.

There are several reasons that children with sleep disordered breathing may end up iron deficient. The first one is that meat is one of the most common sources of dietary iron, but if the nose is blocked, the children have trouble chewing and breathing at the same time, and if the tonsils are big, it can be hard to move meat through the narrow space between the tonsils, and if the tongue is tied, it may be hard to move meat to the back of the throat. All these factors may result in a child that will chew meat, but then spit it out. It is not an aversion to meat, but rather they have worked out that they just can't cope with it. One of the potential by-products of this is that the back of the throat (palate) does not get used to foods of a solid consistency, and the potential consequence of that is the child then develops a sensitive gag reflex because the palate never learnt to deal with more solid things touching it.

The other reason that the iron levels go down though, is that there is a general inflammatory response that occurs in the body when it is subject to chronic intermittent hypoxia. When there is inflammation, the ability of the body to get iron from food into the body is compromised. Studies have shown children with iron deficiency before their tonsils and adenoids are removed, then have normal iron levels after surgery.

There is another reason why having low iron levels is a problem. If you go back to the respiratory system and pulmonary circulation, we talked about how hypoxia causes pulmonary hypertension. Well if you have an iron deficiency, then the pulmonary hypertension is worse again. So it's a bad combination yet again.

Glucose

Glucose is a type of sugar. There are lots of types of sugars, but this is the one the body is geared towards using the most. When sugar is consumed, it is absorbed in the small intestine, hits the blood stream, and as the blood sugar levels rise, this usually triggers a response by the cells of the body to soak up the glucose and use it, or save it for later as an energy source. This absorption of glucose by the cells is usually stimulated by insulin, which comes from a part of the body called the pancreas. If this system does not work properly, then the blood sugar levels in the blood go up, and it they go up too high, we call this diabetes mellitus.

In sleep disordered breathing, there are a multitude of reasons why this system can fall down. For example, an elevation of the body stress hormone, adrenaline, results in a release of sugar from the liver, into the blood, so the muscles are well served by a supply of an energy source. If you are fat, then this results in what is known as insulin resistance, where the insulin is made and released, but it can't stimulate the cells as much as it should, so the sugar hangs around in the blood instead. Intermittent hypoxia also affects liver, fat, and pancreas function. So by all means possible, sugar becomes a growing problem. And if sugar is not consumed, it gets turned in to fat. Which then just makes everything worse.

Lastly, gut bacteria come into the story again. Certain chemicals that they produce seem to impact on the metabolism of glucose. This story just gets worse and worse doesn't it?

Growth hormone and Insulin-like Growth factor 1

In the brain there is a little gland called the pituitary gland. Amongst the many hormones it makes, the most important one is growth hormone. This hormone is crucial for survival as it regulates the activity of every cell of the body. It influences the function of these cells via and intermediate chemical called insulin-like growth factor (abbreviated to IGF), of which there are several types, but the most important type is the first one (IGF-1). And don't let the name fool you- it is called insulin-like because of its chemical structure being similar to insulin, and not because of its affect on the body's sugar metabolism.

In children and adults with upper airway issues, the production of growth hormone is affected. This occurs because the normal brain signals that trigger the release of growth hormone from the pituitary gland are disrupted. The other thing that happens is the levels of IGF-1 are abnormal. The consequence of this is that the growth of the body is affected. This is why children with sleep disordered breathing tend to be shorter than others of the same age. That's the bad news. The good news is that treating the airway obstruction brings these hormone levels back in to balance.

Cholesterol and fat

Fat, in medical terminology, is known as lipids. And while we categorise lipids into many grounds, the main 2 to be aware of are high density lipoproteins (HDL) and low-density lipoproteins (LDL). HDL is what is known as the good fat, and LDL is the bad fat. There are many reasons for having an imbalance in the HDL and LDL levels, including diet, genetics, and obesity. In studies of adults and even children, those who snore have been found to have lower HDL and higher LDL levels. These levels trend towards a normal range once the upper airway obstruction is sorted out. As high LDL and low HDL are risk factors for heart disease and stroke, this is just another important reason to get the breathing optimised.

Catecholamines

These are hormones that result in stimulation of the nervous system and the body in general. We have actually already mentioned a type of hormone that fits this category- adrenaline. - as mentioned above, adrenaline is released at times of stress and excitement. And if the oxygen levels are dropping, this is one such source of excitement that is pathological. So it should come as no surprise by this stage that this is yet another thing that goes wrong in sleep disordered breathing.

Adrenaline has a wide-ranging effect on the body. It causes the heart rate to increase, the strength of each heart beat to increase, the muscles around the arteries contract, and this all leads to the blood pressure going up. So not only do these muscles of the artery contract as a result of increased circulating levels of adrenaline, but also by the direct action of the sympathetic nerves.

It also causes a rise in the blood sugar levels. That's OK if we are in a stressful situation where our muscles are going to be called upon to either fight or take flight, but that's hardly useful when we are trying to sleep.

In terms of measuring the levels of adrenaline, the more interesting things of recent times have been to measure the levels not in the blood, but in the urine also. And the testing confirms elevated levels of this hormone. So, it is not our imagination-there are wide body responses to not being able to breath properly.

Section 3.6 Immunological

As mentioned throughout, one of the things we are aware of in children that have sleep disordered breathing is that they have measurable changes of there being an inflammatory response in their body. It is thought that the chronic intermittent hypoxia is the causative factor that initiates this inflammatory response. In fact, it was finding an elevation in the level of a certain marker of inflammation called C-reactive protein (CRP) in children with sleep apnoea that made us think that we could diagnose significant upper airway obstruction with a simple blood test. Unfortunately, we were not that lucky, as while it can be elevated, it isn't always, and there are other reasons it can be elevated apart from upper airway obstruction.

That finding, though, has led to a much better understanding of how the immune system becomes implicated in sleep disordered breathing. And before we talk about that, don't forget about the gut bacteria contributing to the story with their inflammatory lipopolysaccharides (yeah, OK, I know you probably forgot, that's why I brought it up).

When it comes to measuring markers of inflammation, the most established way is measuring the blood levels of such markers. But there is another way. We can measure certain chemicals in the air we breathe out. This is known as analysis of exhaled breath condensate, and we will get to back to discussing more about that in a moment. It is also worth mentioning that we can measure it in saliva as well, by measuring a chemical called cortisol, which is another body stress hormone.

In terms of blood tests, we can measure the very chemicals that our immune system's white blood cells make. As we are talking literally about hundreds of chemicals, we tend to focus on the more important ones. Amongst the groups of chemicals are 2 main categories, known collectively as leukotrienes and interleukins. And you guessed it; they go up (just like everything else I've mentioned!).

And in terms of exhaled breath concentrate?

Well again we can measure all sorts of things, but the important things we see are a change in the nitric oxide level and elevated levels of leukotrienes. And in adults, when we treat their airway obstruction, these go back to a more normal level. And what is interesting is that it does make a difference as to what the measurements are in adults with sleep apnoea in terms of the time of day that the measurements are taken. The changes seen are evident in the morning, but mostly back to normal by the end of the day.

The changes in adult measurements are also reported in children too.

So, there are definitely things happening at night that result in abnormalities that we can only see at that time. Measurements later throughout the day may give a false sense of reassurance that things are OK.

Section 3.7 Integumentary (skin)

You probably know people spend a fortune on skin care products. OK, not everyone does that. Well it turns out that investing in quality sleep may be a better option. In studies where adults are deliberately limited to 6 hours of sleep, compared to the recommended 8 hours sleep, their skin starts to go pretty bad pretty quickly. And it turns out that the phrase "beauty sleep" really has some meaning. The obvious changes in people deprived of sleep are a worsening of wrinkles and puffy eyes with dark circles around them.

We mentioned cortisol recently as a body stress hormone that we could measure in the saliva. Cortisol acts on the body to break down soft tissue in the skin called collagen and elastin. These two things keep the skin smooth and supple. Cortisol may also result in excess production of oil by the skin pores, which can cause clogging. The elevated cortisol level may also potentially be favourable for the bacteria of the skin to flourish, making the skin worse for the experience. Furthermore, the disrupted sleep affects growth hormone, which important for the skin to rejuvenate itself.

So one of the most important things to do for skin health is getting good night's sleep.

Section 3.8 Musculoskeletal

This entails the bones and muscles of the body. We have talked about the bones of the face already. So let's look at some interesting muscle movements and associated postural changes noted to occur with upper airway obstruction.

So to start with, just to explain, we can look at how muscles function by placing a small probe into the muscle and measuring its activity. This is called an EMG. And there are studies where we have looked at the activity in the tongue, lips, muscles of the face and jaws, and muscles of the neck in those that snore and those that don't. We have even done it in those that have tongue ties and grind their teeth. And we have also measured it in the muscles of breathing. And the findings are very interesting, to say the least!

To understand what we are about to talk about, think about the facial expressions someone put on when they go to lift something heavy- they draw a breath in, hold it tight, their eyes are wide open, and their mouth pouts out as they lift. What they are doing is bracing themselves for the upcoming effort, and recruiting their whole body to allow them to lift the weight. So it is not just the arms doing the work, it's the co-ordination of the legs, torso, arms and so forth to accomplish the lift. Now keep that mental image in mind as we look at what happens to the muscles in the territory of where there is an airway problem.

So let's start with tongue tie. Now just to remind you, this is where the tongue is held down to the lower part of the bottom of the mouth. As a result, it has to work harder to push food to the back of the throat. What is interesting in this regard is that the muscles of the lips and cheeks are also recruited to help move things along in such cases. And it was not just in swallowing that these changes were evident. In actions such as clenching the teeth, swallowing, and even kissing, the muscle activity in those with tongue ties is different. And once the tongue tie is released, after a couple of months, the extra muscle activity goes back to normal.

So let's go to sleep disordered breathing.

Grinding the teeth at night is known as sleep bruxism. What it is, basically, is the muscles of the jaw pulling the lower jaw up tightly, and then moving the jaw from sided to side, causing the teeth to crunch against each other. Not only does this result in a terrible noise but sometimes the teeth can get worn down and crack under the pressure of the muscle contraction.

Now in truth, nobody knows why exactly this happens, but as time has gone by, the historical perspective that it is due to "stress" is being challenged by the better understanding of the things that happen at night when there is intermittent hypoxia. Now we are certain that psychological stress does indeed cause some people to grind their teeth. But here is another one of those vicious circles, because, having sleep disordered breathing has been shown to increase your levels of anxiety. So that makes things a bit complicated.

So what do we know about sleep bruxism and upper airway obstruction? Well we know that in children that grind their teeth, for those that have an airway problem that is then treated, close to 80% of them stop grinding their teeth. And adults? Well for adults who have has sleep apnoea diagnosed, there are studies that show treatment with either a special mouth guard or a special breathing mask (called CPAP- we will come to that later), they too often stop grinding their teeth. In fact, the recognition of the relationship between airway problems and grinding in teeth in adults is now such that experts are starting to recommend assessing for a breathing problem before managing the teeth grinding. In other words, addressing the potential cause.

And whilst grinding the teeth is an obvious thing for other people to hear, or for dentists to notice, it turns out that even minimal extra jaw movements are evident with a study showing that intermittent hypoxia can result in micro-movements of the low jaw. So it is possible that bruxism is an extreme manifestation of the lower oxygen levels brought about by upper airway obstruction. We have so much to learn still!

Mouth breathing

The changes brought about by nasal versus mouth breathing were discussed in the context of the effect on oxygen levels. But there is more to the story. In a study on adults who were either nose breathers or mouth breathers, they measured which muscles they were using to breathe with. Now when we breathe, there is a big muscle at the base of the chest called the diaphragm that pulls the lungs down. Furthermore, on the side walls of the chest, between the ribs, there are muscles that pull the ribs to expand the chest outwards. There are also muscles in the neck that pull the ribs up too. And they found differences in how these muscles were activated with the route of breathing between the mouth breathing versus nose breathing groups. In a nutshell, nose breathing was more functional, with greater engagement of the diaphragm.

Another thing that happens with mouth breathing is that the activation of the neck muscles may result in changes in head posture. In a study of mouth breathing versus nasal breathing children, they did find that such a change in head posture occurs, with the head being pulled forwards.

In terms of changes in facial muscle activity, again in mouth breathers, the research finds changes in the activity of muscles around the chin, and even the eyes themselves. It's pretty incredible isn't it?

Section 3.8 Genitourinary system

In this section I am going to mention reproductive health but focus more so upon bed wetting. Although these functions are quite separate, anatomically they are related and hence grouped together.

Male fertility

We know that obstructive sleep apnoea in male adults can lead to erectile dysfunction. In a study in mice, it also reduced the motility of sperm. Such mice were less likely to result in impregnation of their female counterparts. So not only do men have problems with their ability to perform, they are essentially, to be blunt, more likely to be shooting blanks also.

Bed wetting

It is normal for children to wet the bed- at least to a point. At some stage in a child's (and parent's) life, it becomes frustrating, and a source of embarrassment. In children that wet the bed we tend to be proactive if it occurs beyond the suggested ages of what may be considered acceptable and normal (and this is argued to be anywhere between 5-8 years of age). There are several reasons a child may wet the bet beyond this range, and having sleep disordered breathing is certainly one such reason, but there are a host of factors at play, so let's go through them.

First up, let's visit the stress response that results in a release of adrenaline. This puts the blood pressure up, increasing the pressure of the blood as it goes through the kidneys. This can result in an increased amount of fluid being filtered through the kidney by virtue of the increased pressure. There are other compensatory mechanisms that may mean this potential effect is not a big player in the game, but every little drop adds up.

Intermittent hypoxia induces an inflammatory response. It turns out this does affect the kidney. In fact in animal studies it has been shown to damage the kidneys. This also makes sense from a clinical point of view, as we know that in adults with both sleep apnoea and kidney failure, those patients' kidney function deteriorates faster than those who do not have sleep apnoea.

Hormonal changes

Now apart from adrenaline, there are some other hormones that are abnormal in their levels in those with upper airway obstruction. The 2 of relevance in bed wetting are called "anti-diuretic hormone" (ADH) and "brain natriuretic peptide" (BNP). In children with SDB, ADH is decreased and BNP is increased.

Now the job of ADH is to make the kidney produce less urine. The job of BNP is to make more urine. BNP is released more when the heart is under a lot of pressure. As there is so much going on with the blood pressure and heart function in children, this leads to an elevation on BNP, to try and settle things down.

So we have an elevation of one hormone that increases urine production at the same time as having a decrease in a hormone that makes less urine. So the net effect is you make a lot more urine. So this means the bladder fills up with more urine that it may otherwise do so through the course of the night. And there is a limit as to how much a bladder can hold on to.

As an aside, guess what happens in children that have surgery for their airway problems? These hormone levels go back to normal.

So that's the production of urine taken care of. Now how about being able to hold it in?

The bladder is basically a muscular bag. It collects urine from the kidneys, and when it gets to a certain filling size, the stretch of the walls of the bladder triggers a signal to say it is time to void. This signal can be over-ridden, which is why you can "hold on" but also way sometimes you are busting. In animal studies of the muscle activity of the bladder, it has been found that the ability to hold on is reduced. This is called detrusor instability. This happens due to reduced oxygen levels causing a build up of certain chemicals in the muscle that then changes how this muscle behaves. The other thing that triggers it to empty is an increase in the muscle tone of the bladder caused by adrenaline- yep, that thing again.

Section 4. Investigations of people who snore

The focus of this section is to explain the types of tests that can be used to assess for airway problems. Whilst the previous discussions have talked about lots of medical problems that can occur due to upper airway obstruction (diabetes, for example), we are not going to talk about the tests for those other conditions.

In terms of tests and investigations, there is a lot that has been alluded to thus far, but now we are going to go into far more detail on things that are used in clinical practice. Many things mentioned so far belong to fields of research rather than mainstream clinical assessment. The reasons for this vary, from some things are just impractical, to others are very expensive, to some are just not good enough to be suited for reliable clinical assessment.

In terms of the tests we will talk about, we will discuss how they work, and what their limitations are.

Thyroid function test

In adults, this is the most important test to have done. The thyroid gland is involved in regulating the body's metabolism. And there are many reasons why this gland can stop working. The symptoms of an underperforming thyroid gland are exactly the same as obstructive sleep apnoea. A simple blood test can assess for this. By doing so, treatment with a simple thyroid supplement can re-establish the thyroid gland hormone levels to normal. And for some people, this is the only treatment they require.

Acoustic rhinometry

This is a test of the nose, to see if it is blocked or clear. The way it works is a bit like how bats navigate- a sound wave is sent in to the nose by a probe and a sensor measures what bounces back. The more that bounces back, the more the nose is blocked. Furthermore, the time taken for the sound wave to travel in and then bounce back allows calculations on where the sound bounced from and gives an idea of where and by how much the nose may be blocked.

Now while this sounds good in theory, remember that the nose can change where and when it is blocked due to the nasal cycle. The problem with this test is that it does not tell us why the nose is blocked. So it has been used by some just to demonstrate to patients that there is a problem with their nose physically, even if the patient feels things are OK. The challenge for those with a chronically blocked nose is that patients may be so used to having a blocked nose that they don't realise how bad things are. In practical terms though, this sort of test is more interesting and usefuls for research rather than being of any real practical use in normal clinical situations.

Pharyngometry

Just like we can use a sound wave to measure the nose, we can do the same in the throat. Since the proper name for the throat is pharynx, we now come to pharyngometry. Again, this is more of interest in research fields than clinical application, though there is possibly a role for it in one instance and that is in adults with upper airway obstruction who are having treatment with a special mouth guard-like device made by a dentist, called a mandibular advancement splint. This device works by drawing the bottom jaw forwards, which puts tension through the muscles of the throat, and in some cases this will then open the throat up. Pharyngometry is a way for dentists to measure the degree of opening of the pharynx when the device is used. It is not a perfect modality, and only measures a patient's airway when they are awake, but it does provide some useful feedback to help guide the design and setting of the splint in some patients.

Radiological imaging

Another way of assessing the airway, apart from looking at the patient, is to take certain x-rays. Now there are 3 main categories of imaging that have been utilised in assessing the airway- plain films, CT scans, and MRI scans. So let's go through these in detail.

Plain film x-rays are the most basic of images that can be done. They are basically a snap shot taken from one side through to the other, and all the structures are represented on the image produced. Unfortunately, all these structures overlap each other, so the image produced is blurred. That makes interpretation of the images rather difficult. In terms of the main thing that people have tried to look at, it is the size of the adenoids that has been the main area of interest. Now this makes sense, as the only way of physically assessing the size of the adenoids in a patient is to use a telescope that is passed through the nose. Now truth be told, this is usually actually relatively easy, even in children, but it is the domain of an Ear, Nose, and Throat specialist, so that somewhat limits that option. However, just because that is a limited option does not justify alternatives if those alternatives are not very good in themselves.

So how good is plain film x-ray for measuring the size of the adenoids? In short, not very good at all. Studies of patients who have had an ENT look inside the nose, and assessed the size of the adenoids on direct examination, when compared to what the x-rays suggested, reveals that the x-rays were too inaccurate to commend them. Despite that, the method of assessment is still in common use, meaning a radiation dose to a child with no definite certainty that the result is correct.

Plain film x-rays have also been used to allow certain specialists to look at the position of the bones and make some measurements of the relationship of certain bones to others. This helps guide them in the decision making process of certain types of jaw surgery. That's about it though for plain film x-rays.

The other type of x-ray that involves a radiation is what is called a CT scan (or a CAT scan in some places). Now the pictures generated by a CT scan are certainly much clearer than a plain film, and with the software today, gives a lot of information too. But again, it is a radiation dose, and it needs to be questioned if that is a good idea purely to assess the adenoids.

The third type of imaging is called an MRI. There is no radiation with this technique. The problem is that it takes 20-45 minutes and requires the patient to stay still the whole time. Needless to say that's a pretty big ask for a child. Furthermore, the information we get is more in the category of interesting than useful for clinical management.

So as appealing as using body imaging technology is, they are no where near the same value as a direct look at things.

Sleep endoscopy

An endoscope is a special telescope that can look inside the body. A technique that has been developed involves patients having an anaesthetic to induce a state of simulated sleep, and during this time, an endoscope is passed in to the throat, to try and see what is going on. This method has some advantages, in that it allows the assessor to view the airway when the muscles are in a relaxed state, which is comparable to certain phases of sleep, but has a disadvantage that the patient must be lying on their back during this assessment, and other body positions can not be assessed in terms of the status of the airway. This last point is important, as some people do not sleep on their back and also, some people only get problems when they are on their back. Furthermore, there is no accurate or precise means of knowing if the right amount of anaesthetic is being given to simulate the relaxation of sleep. So whilst very popular in some clinics, it is important to understand the limitations of such assessments, especially given that it involves the administration of anaesthetic medications.

Sleep studies

These are considered the gold standard for measuring how badly the airway becomes obstructed. Unfortunately, they do not indicate which part of the airway is blocked, and do not indicate what treatment options (which are all discussed in the next section) are best suited for a patient.

Sleep studies come in different shapes and sizes. As is often the case in many situations, the more information you have the better. So in an ideal world, a sleep study would be a standardised test with well recognised monitoring that is offered in every setting. However, for practical reasons, this can't be offered to everybody. As a result, there is a range of test options, and this adds to the confusion as to the validity of sleep studies.

So what do sleep studies measure?

The most comprehensive of studies will measure all of the following:

- time spent asleep
- movement of air with each breath
- chest wall movement
- inner chest cavity pressure level
- brain wave patterns
- snoring intensity
- oxygen levels
- heart rate and rhythm

- movements of the jaw
- blood pressure
- body position

These measurements all require special sensors to be worn whilst asleep. This is the next criticism on the validity of sleep studies-some people just find these all very uncomfortable, and may not get the best night's sleep. The other issue, potentially, is that people change their behaviours when they have sleep studies, in particular decreasing their usual amount of alcohol consumed. This behavioural modification is a good thing, but if limited to the night of the sleep study, a normal study may give false reassurance if their normal alcohol consumption is such that it results in airway obstruction.

So let's go through the sensors and monitors involved in a sleep study, and why each one of them is important.

Breathing monitor

This is a simple monitor that measures airflow in and out of your mouth/nose. It also measures the volume of airflow, so it can pick up when the airflow stops, but also when it decreases below a normal average volume. To remind you, an apnoea is a cessation of airflow completely, and a hypopnoea is a reduction in the normal volume of airflow by at least 50%.

This monitoring is the most important part of a sleep study. The great thing about them is not only does it measure the breathing, but it can record the duration of an impaired breathing episode, and with this information, a calculation can be made on the number of events per hour, plus the average duration of events. This can be quite helpful for explaining to patients how bad they are. Some people record events that are longer than their ability to hold their breath whilst awake- which is quite scary really.

Chest wall movement

Whilst the breathing monitor can pick up airflow, if the airflow is reduced, it does not know if this was because you were trying to breathe but couldn't (obstructive apnoea) or whether the airflow changed because the brain did not tell the body to take a breath (central apnoea). That is where the chest wall monitor comes into play. By measuring the movement of the chest wall, and matching it to airflow, this will help differentiate between either a cessation or reduction in airflow due to either obstruction or lack of effort.

Inner chest cavity pressure level

Bearing in mind that the chest wall monitor can measure the presence of an effort or not to breathe, it can not measure the intensity of this effort. This is a really important concept to think about. To help understand this, think about this for a moment: if there is an obstruction to the breathing, if you put more effort in to breathing, the breathing monitor will record a normal breath, and the chest wall monitor will confirm an effort was made. But having to work extra hard just to get a normal breath in, is not the same as breathing normally. This is where a monitor measuring the pressure level within the chest cavity itself can provide some very important information. Unfortunately this is one of the least used monitors in sleep studies, which means a potential under-representation of the severity of someone's airway issues. This is particularly the case in children.

So why is this measurement rarely done?

Basically it is because of all the measurements, it is the only one that could be considered invasive. The monitor for this needs to physically sit inside the chest wall itself. Now before you start to think about some sort of probe being inserted by stabbing you through the ribs, there is some good news! The practical way of doing this measurement is having the monitor attached to the end of a tube, and this tube is passed back through the nose, down the throat, and in to the oesophagus. Now this is entirely possible, but children are not going to be keen on it, and many adults aren't either. So this is one problem of sleep studies that is unavoidable in unco-operative patients.

Brain wave patterns

The brain is able to be monitored for its rhythms and patterns. This is really helpful because in sleep, there are different stages. And there are differences in breathing, muscle activity, and all sorts of other things that impact on the measurements otherwise being made. So measuring the brain activity provides an important context for the results of other measurements. The other good thing is that it is pretty easy to measure, with some stickers placed on the head that have a lead that goes in to the monitoring device.

Snoring intensity

This is pretty easy- it is just a microphone. It's actually quite important, as some people refuse to believe that they snore. It's also important because not every one with sleep apnoea snores. So the lack of snoring does not necessarily equate to a lack of breathing problems. In simple terms, you snore because there is obstruction. But for there to be snoring, there needs to be airflow- some people are so obstructed that there is not even enough airflow to generate a snoring noise.

Oxygen levels

The whole crux of upper airway obstruction is the intermittent drop in oxygen levels. You may recall we referred to this as intermittent hypoxia. Now measuring the oxygen levels is pretty straight forward, with a simple probe placed on the finger, toe, or even the ear lobe able to measure the oxygen levels. One problem though is that these sensors work on average levels rather than absolute levels. As a result, a quick dip in the oxygen level may not register, as it gets averaged out and ignored when compared to the rest of the time where the oxygen levels are OK. So it's handy to know if someone is really bad, but it is also important to be mindful of limitations.

Heart rate and rhythm

When the oxygen levels drop, this sets off an emergency signal in the brain. One of the consequences of this is that the heart is stimulated to beat faster. This stimulation can sometimes trigger an abnormal response, where the heart goes into overdrive. Specifically, the heart can start beating irregularly. An irregular heart beat is called an arrhythmia. And the most common type of arrhythmia is something called atrial fibrillation. Some people end up needing drugs or even special interventional heart procedures to stop their heart behaving this way. It is now recognised that identifying sleep apnoea as a cause of the irregular heart beat is very important as treating the underlying cause makes a lot of sense.

Movements of the jaw

As mentioned above, there are different stages of sleep. And muscle activity varies between these stages of sleep. In some people, when their oxygen levels drop down, the stimulated brain may activate some of the muscles around the jaw, and this may then result in grinding and clenching of the teeth. This only happens in certain stages of sleep. So it is again helpful to measure the muscle activity of the muscles around the jaw and to also match this up with the stage of sleep. As this muscle activity is only of passing interest to medical doctors (but of great interest to dentists), it unfortunately is also on the list of measurements that may not necessarily be done as part of a sleep study. That is a shame, as it only needs some stickers applied to the face to monitor the muscle activity.

Blood pressure

It is now thought that it is possible that changes in blood pressure in children results in having high blood pressure as an adult. For some people, their blood pressure goes quite high if they have airway obstruction. Furthermore, it may be that for some people, their blood pressure goes highest at night, during these obstructive episodes. So from that point of view, measuring the blood pressure is really important at night. As an aside, speaking as an ENT specialist for a moment, one of the reasons some people get blood noses is because they have high blood pressure, and interestingly, some people get blood noses only at night- these people may well have airway obstruction at night, so it is something I am always on the look out for. Measuring the blood pressure is really easy, so it is usually done routinely.

Body position

For those of us with smart phones, we know that is we tip it sideways, the screen will rotate, and they can also help monitor our route of travel. This technology is also applied in sleep studies, with a simple monitor strapped on that records the position of the body. This is really important, as some people only obstruct in certain body positions. Given this is the case, some people can have their airway obstruction managed simply by wearing devices that encourage a certain body position. So knowing about the relationship of body position to times of obstruction is a really important as it helps in deciding on how to manage patients.

How do we use all of this information?

Well there is a complex answer and an easy answer. I am in to easy answers. In doing so, please note that the following numbers applies to adults, and not children.

The total time spent asleep is important, as that is our reference range for calculating the average number of events that happen per hour of sleep time. A person with normal sleep habits sleeps between 6-8 hours per night.

The first thing we want to know is how many times did the person have trouble breathing through the night. To do this we want to know about the number of apnoeas, and the number of hypopneas. Remember, an apnoea in adults is considered to be an event of stopping breathing for at least 10 seconds and a hypopnoea is a reduction in airflow by at least 50%. The number of apnoeas and hypopnoeas are added together, and this number is then divided by the total sleep time to determine the average number of events per hour

This is known as the Apnoea-Hypopnea Index, or AHI for short. The normal AHI in an adult is less than 5.

A possibly more useful number incorporates the number of episodes of breathing reduction with another type of breathing measurement that is known as a Respiratory Effort Related Arousal (RERA to add to the list of abbreviations). In simple terms, this is a short (few seconds) period or arousal that follows on from a partial occlusion of the airway. Using this measurement, we can add these events to the apnoeas and hypopnoeas and then divide this total by the duration of sleep, and we then come to another index, known as the respiratory disturbance index (abbreviated to RDI). The normal RDI is less than 5.

As stated throughout this book, oxygen is really important. Oxygen makes up about 21% of the atmospheric air. It is the most important thing we need, and we need a constant supply. If the oxygen levels in the blood decrease, then we call this a desaturation. Decreased oxygen levels means that the heart needs to work harder. In adults, we can measure the oxygen levels and then set a limit for how low the desaturations are before we start to worry. We can then tally up these episodes of significant desaturation. In adults we calculate an index known as the oxygen desaturation index (ODI). This is the average number of times the oxygen levels decrease by 4% or more per hour of sleep time. The normal range, you guessed it, is less than 5.

Sleep follows a pattern. And this brings us to an important element of sleep, and that is the quality of sleep. One of the big divisions of sleep patterns is in to REM versus non-REM sleep. REM stands for rapid eye movement. The REM stage of sleep is very important as we believe it is where most of the benefits of a good night sleep occur. It is also the stage when people have their dreams. The normal range of REM, as a percentage of the total sleep time is 15-30%.

By bringing together the array of diverse measurements, we can then synthesise an understanding of the patient's sleep and breathing patterns, with an indication of how bad they are, and whether there are measurable impacts upon oxygen levels, heart function, blood pressure, and brain function, for example. However, as stated, this only tells us how bad the obstruction is, not which part of the airway is obstructing. That is why a sleep study is not the only aspect of airway assessment, as it makes no sense to advice on treatment options without knowing about the cause of the problem in the first place. So on that basis, we shall move forwards to the next section, which is all about treatment.

Section 5. Treatment of the causes of obstruction

Well it has been a long journey to get to this point, but with a simple problem like restricting the ability to breathe there is literally a disaster of consequences through out the whole body. So, we need to fix this problem!

There are a mass of treatment and management options. There is a difference between the meaning of the word "treatment" and "management". We should be pedantic and use words specific to their meaning. So when we say treatment, technically we mean something that fixes the problem to some degree, and when we talk about management, we mean that we alleviate the problem with an intervention, but it is still there unless that intervention is used consistently. This may sound confusing, but think about a broken arm bone- the treatment is a plaster cast (and time), but part of the management is pain killers. Now pain killers do not fix a broken bone, but they sure do help, so we call it management rather than treatment. So basically, treatment is about fixing the problem, and management is about making the associated symptoms (but not the cause) better.

In its most basic form, we can divide treatment and management in to the following (with a comment in bracket indicating whether this falls into treatment or management):

- Nothing (Neither treatment nor management)

- Physical therapy and lifestyle modification [eg. diet and exercise] (Treatment)
- Medication (Treatment)
- Surgery (Treatment)
- Weight loss (Treatment)
- Wearing a night time mask that allows air to be pumped into the throat – this is called CPAP (Management)
- Appliance that sits inside the mouth, and holds the airway open by holding the jaw in a certain position (Management) or a device that over time physically stretches the bones of the middle of the face outwards to create more room [known as expansion] (Treatment)

So using this framework, let's go through these things in more detail.

Physical therapy

- Diet, exercise, weight loss

It is well known that we are leading more sedentary lifestyles and eating foods that have been heavily processed. Which ever way you look at it, the consequences of our modern-day living is that as a community, we are getting fat. And being fat is bad for your health, and this includes your sleep quality. It is well documented that being overweight and obese significantly increases your chances of having airway obstruction at night. So it is time for many people to take responsibility for their own health and take the initiative of improving their level of physical activity and moderating what they eat, and how much they eat. By doing so, the weight will start to drop off, and amongst the many benefits this confers, the propensity to airway obstruction also dissipates.

With so much to be gained from losing weight, a reasonable question is why doctors do not focus on this more or advocate such lifestyle modifications? Part of it, to be honest, is that it is not a great focus of ours (but it should be), and the other part of it, realistically, is that such changes are better to come from within and are more likely to be acted upon if the patient makes the deliberate decision to make changes, and carries out with an action plan to achieve those changes, than any amount of general advice ever will achieve.

Having said that, here are some very simple suggestions that many people could adopt, and by doing so, they would alter their diet ever so slightly, but it would make a big difference. So here goes: when it comes to drinks, drink more water in preference to drinking fruit juice and soft drinks, and when it comes to food, eat more fruit and vegetables and less fast foods and processed foods. If you look at this advice, it is pretty easy to follow, but some people will find even this too hard, and there in lies the problem for those people.

The other aspect from a lifestyle modification point of view is looking at alcohol intake, and sleep routines.

Alcohol is an easy topic to cover- in a nutshell, it should be used in moderation for enjoyment and pleasure rather than as a staple part of the diet or lifestyle. It also is best not to be consuming it within 2 hours of going to sleep. Lastly, it is a lot of calories that come with it and this is not good for your weight.

Sleep hygiene is a problem of modern living. The best way to get your body clock back in to synchronisation with its natural rhythm is to go out camping, avoiding artificial light, and living by the sun coming up and going down. It is thought that after about a week, things will be more in line with where they need to be. Realistically though, we rely on alarm clocks to rouse us from our sleep- which is actually interrupting our sleep, then we use coffee to get us going, and at the end of the day, we stay up later due to artificial lighting allowing us to do so, and we engage our eyes and brain with TV screens and computers and phones, resulting in abnormal brain activity at the end of the day that flows on to the night, only for the next alarm to then rouse us to do it all again.

- Exercises for the throat

Apart from general body exercise to help with weight loss, there are specific exercises that can be helpful for improving the strength and tone of the muscles around the throat. There is a general word that is applied to the whole range of exercises to deal with the function of the mouth, tongue, and throat muscles which is "myofunctional".

This is a whole new area of interest for those health practitioners involved in managing children and adults with upper airway obstruction. Presently, it is an area of both research and debate, with some healthy scepticism thrown in to the mix. But slowly but surely, the research is coming out showing favourable benefits of such therapy.

Now, as many people who have taken out gym memberships will know, things can get boring after a while, so there have been some lateral thinking people out there that have done some pretty interesting research on different methods of getting people to perform exercises for their throat. In particular, there has been benefit shown in two most unusual and peculiar of circumstances....

Firstly, and this is an Australian flavour to the topic, there has been research in adults with obstructive sleep apnoea graded as being moderate who were taught to play, of all things, the Australian Aboriginal didgeridoo. After 3 months of daily playing of this instrument, the study population had another sleep study, with the results compared to their original findings. Quite impressive was the fact that these patients had better results for having played the instrument.

A second area of interest in encouraging patients to perform exercises is engaging them in singing lessons. Once again, under professional tutelage, patients who immersed themselves in the ins and outs of using their throat, voice box, and breathing patterns in the right way also improved in terms of their sleep study results.

I suggest patients get some balloons and blow them up at night. I have no scientific evidence that this works, but it is an easy thing for people to do.

Despite the evidence being there, unfortunately many adult patients are not even told about these scientific studies and, furthermore, these adjunct therapies are left to the wayside. In fact, all too often a lifelong prescription of a breathing mask is made without patients even being fully examined, denying them the opportunity to know about all of the management choices that are on offer.

Medications

In situations where there is a process contributing to upper airway obstruction that is amenable to simple medications, then it is important that patients are offered the opportunity to have these trialled. The particular conditions related to upper airway obstruction are reflux and allergic rhinitis.

- Anti-Reflux therapy

Reflux is the condition where stomach contents will come up to the back of the throat, via the oesophagus. In simple terms, there are 3 ways of medicating this condition- the first is reducing the acid content of the stomach, and the second is improving the motility of the stomach so it empties its contents more effectively, so things are not hanging around in the stomach for too long, and the third is to ingest something that sits as a protective coating over the lining of the throat and oesophagus. By far, the first option is the most utilised.

Before using medication though, the first thing that should be done in patients with reflux is addressing the diet and lifestyle factors that contribute to the problem. When it comes to diet, the things that are known to induce reflux are caffeine containing substances (tea, coffee, chocolate, soft drinks), fatty foods, spicy foods, alcohol, and acid foods (such as tomatoes). From a lifestyle point of view, eating too close to going to bed is not a good idea, and smoking isn't that great either. Some people find that elevating the head end of their bed is useful too.

If you are on other medications for other conditions, some of these can make reflux worse, so it is important to have a doctor review your therapies if this is the case.

For some patients, even though they do everything suggested, they still have reflux that is so bad, that surgery on the stomach to tighten up where the oesophagus enters in to it is the only thing that stops the reflux from happening.

- Nasal allergy

There are many medications for the congestion that comes with a bout of hayfever. By far, as a general comment, nasal sprays are much better for clearing the nose up than are oral medications. In terms of oral tablets, the most common ones in use are known as antihistamines. These are good for a runny nose, itchy eyes, and sneezing, but do little to settle down the nasal swelling and hence improve the obstruction.

In terms of nasal sprays, there are 3 main groups to mention. The first are non-medicated saline (salt water) sprays. These are a good general option, as they have no side effects, but as a stand alone option, usually won't do very much. The next group of sprays some people reach for are known as decongestants. This is a bad option. These sprays are addictive, and truth be known, play a minimal role in the practice of ENT specialists. Which brings us to the main group of nasal sprays worthy of use, and these are steroid based sprays.

Now for some people, the word "steroid" conjures up all sorts of ideas, but it is important to keep everything in context. Just like there are different sorts of antibiotics, there are different sorts of steroids. The types used in nasal sprays are not the sort used by those who abuse their bodies in the name of muscle or body building. These steroids are anti-inflammatory in their action, and work much better than antihistamines because they do everything that antihistamines do plus they reduce the swelling within the nose, opening up the airway. It is important to note that there are certain ones approved for use in children, and some that are only approved for use in adults, so it is important to get good advice.

Weight loss

Losing weight can be particularly difficult, but even more so in those that have sleep apnoea.

Whilst the usual basics of diet and exercise apply, there are some genuine things that interfere with this being successful. Firstly, having sleep apnoea means you may be tired during the day. So people just don't have the energy or motivation to undertake physical activity. The next problem is that for those that are overweight, their joints may be starting to ache and become arthritic simply because of the extra weight they have to support through the day. The last thing from an exercise point of view is that if the heart and lungs are already straining to keep up with things, then the added burden of exercise may not be so easy, and this will limit their functioning activity.

The next challenge is diet. And in this regard, there is another vicious circle to contend with. Studies have been done that shows that the parts of the brain that regulate appetite are dysfunctional in those with sleep apnoea. Specifically, the brain becomes geared towards craving high calorie foods. It is hard to be sure why this is the case, but one school of thought is that the stress responses brought about by obstructive sleep apnoea results in an altered metabolic demand, and the brain is tricked in to thinking the body needs more energy. The other thing that happens is that there are a range of body hormone changes that are geared towards preserving fat stores. The good news is that with effort, as the weight drops, these hormonal changes start to reverse, so it does get easier, but it takes a while.

For some people, their weight is such a problem, that surgery is their only option. The results from surgery in the short term can be quite good, but unless true behavioural changes come from within, then such measures may only have a limited long-term benefit.

Surgery for upper airway obstruction

OK, now we are getting to where the value of an ENT surgeon is at its greatest, and that is by physically addressing the airway obstruction. Just as I worked through the points of airway obstruction systematically, from top down, so too will I structure the discussion on surgery. All of the operations to be discussed are performed by ENT surgeons, except for the last one (jaw surgery), where it is mostly done by maxillofacial surgeons.

- Nasal obstruction- septum, turbinates, adenoids, polyps

The crooked nasal septum can be made straight again with surgery. Depending on the severity of the deformity determines the amount of surgery involved. Most of the time, the surgery is done internally, but if the septum is severely deformed, than an approach involving a small cut under the nose, to gain access may be necessary. Sometimes the outer bones of the bridge of the nose are also crooked, and these can be straightened up at the time also. It is now thought to be OK to operate on a growing child's nasal septum, as long as the methods used are conservative rather than aggressive.

Either in conjunction with septal surgery, or alone, the inferior nasal turbinates can be operated upon. There are several different types of operations for the turbinates, and it is important to understand the differences when discussing this with your specialist. The first is called turbinate cautery. This involves applying heat to the nasal turbinate soft tissue lining, with the intention of inducing scar tissue. This scar tissue contracts to shrink the turbinate size. This works OK, but often not for much longer than about 6-12 months, so it is probably best for little children where access is a problem, knowing that it will buy some time for them to grow, and if the nasal obstruction recurs, then they will be bigger and alternative surgical options will be possible.

The next type of inferior turbinate surgery involves the use of an instrument that melts the tissue away, but not with heat but rather by turning the soft tissue into mush. It does this using technology called radio-frequency ablation. This method seems to work quite well, but again, the results may not last forever, with studies suggesting the nose may block up again 2-5 years down the track. So again, not a bad option for children where access for other types of surgery is an issue.

The last category of surgery for the inferior turbinates to be mentioned is known as micro-debrider assisted inferior turbinoplasty. In simple terms, a micro-debrider is a special device that can remove soft tissue by virtue of it having a small rotating blade- think or is as being a bit like an electric shaver. By removing the soft tissue, this exposes the underlying bone of the inferior turbinate. This bone is very small, and easily removed. By doing so, the space inside the nose is significantly increased. When performing this operation, some of the tissue of the inferior turbinate is preserved, as it is an important part of the nose for the purposes of humidifying the air we breathe in.

The adenoids sit in the back of the nose, They may be removed as a stand alone procedure or in combination with other ENT operations. The most common types of things it is combined with is any of the nasal surgery discussed above, with tonsil removal, and/or with the insertion of special tubes in to the ear drum called grommets (or ventilation tubes, or pressure equalising tubes). As the adenoids sit at the back of the throat, behind the nose, they are not visible to normal examination. There are, however, 2 ways of visualising the adenoids at the time of surgery- either looking through the nose with a nasal endoscope, or looking through the mouth with either an endoscope that can look around corners, or even easier, a mirror.

Now at this point you may be surprised to learn that the most common method for removing adenoids is to not even bother looking at all. In fact, this is how I was first taught. This method involves opening the mouth, using a special scraping device called an adenotome (or adenoid curette), and putting this device blindly in to the back of the nose and shaving the adenoids out, and then feeling with your finger to see if it seems like the adenoids are all out. It may not surprise you that when studies of this technique have been done, that it does not actually work very well. In fact one study showed that about 70% of the time, adenoids were left behind. Despite us knowing this, this technique is still being taught.

Fortunately there are places where they have progressed beyond blind techniques, and using either a mirror or a telescope, the adenoids are removed either under vision, or the area is assessed at the completion of the operation, to ensure that the adenoids are adequately removed. I am a real advocate for patients understanding that there are different ways of doing operations and those different methods in different surgeon's hands do yield different results.

- Tonsils

The tonsils sit on the side wall of the throat. There are different ways of removing them, and this in itself does not really matter, except in the case of a carbon dioxide laser. The use of such a laser was quite popular at one stage. It is probably the worst option to have ever been entertained, as it is very destructive. Having said that, this destruction makes it perfect for removing tonsils that have turned cancerous, so be mindful that there are no absolutes, and that everything has its place.

For the mainstay, either surgical dissection, radiofrequency dissection, or cautery dissection are the 3 most common approaches these days. Each has the pros and cons, but the important factor is the experience of the surgeon with their technique, and their complication rate. The main complication is bleeding after tonsil removal. Now as per any sort of operation, a little bit of bleeding after is normal. It is when a little bit turns in to a lot that a trip back to hospital is necessary. Most of the time, a lot of bleeding will settle down, but sometimes it requires another operation to sort things out. It varies, but it is considered within the realm of acceptable if the rate of post-operative bleeding that requires another operation to control the haemorrhage is no more than 4% of a surgeon's cases. Just to share, my rate at the time of writing this book is less than 1%. And I even do this operation now as a day surgery procedure most of the time, reflecting my confidence in the techniques I use.

- Tongue tie

The most common types of tongue tie are relatively easy to fix. Whilst people argue over the method, the truth is that in experienced hands, whatever technique they use is the one that they find they are best at. Most of these can be done under local anaesthetic, but some are quite tricky and best done with the patient asleep.

- Palate

We can shorten the palate if it is too long, stiffen it if it is too floppy, and relocate it to a more forward position if it is sitting too far back. Not too tricky hey?!

- Lingual tonsils

Now these are tricky. There are tricky firstly because they sit down the throat, and gaining access to them is not the easiest. The second reason they are tricky is because there is really not an obvious boundary between where these lingual tonsils finish, and the tongue starts. Furthermore, the operation tends to lend itself to bleeding, and this can be tricky to stop at times. Due to these difficulties, it is one area where robotic assisted surgery is being explored as an option. In the meantime, fortunately, this operation is rarely needed as medication such as antibiotics and anti-reflux treatments shrink these lingual tonsils down.

- Jaw surgery

This is usually performed by maxillofacial surgeons. It is surgery whereby either the top or bottom (or both) jaws are surgically separated, and then repositioned. The repositioning is a movement of the jaws forward. This creates more space internally. It is usually reserved for adults that have developmentally deficient facial bones.

That is a brief summary of surgery options for children and adults with upper airway obstruction. Now we come to alternative options, and these are offered by those who are not surgically inclined.

CPAP

This stands for continuous positive airway pressure. In simple terms, this is what most people equate to understanding as being the mask that is worn at night. In simple terms, this works by pumping air in to the throat all of the time, to keep it open. Think of the concept of blowing up a balloon and keeping your mouth over the balloon to keep it inflated. Well it is the same sort of thing, except in reverse- the patient is now the balloon. These sorts of masks come in all sorts of shapes and sizes. In the mainstay, they are used in adults far more commonly than in children.

CPAP is often prescribed without patients being examined by an ENT. Probably the most common problem patients with CPAP have is the discomfort of the mask, especially if high pressures are needed to maintain the airway. While CPAP may help people at night, it fails to treat any day time obstruction. I think every patient that is a candidate for CPAP should be assessed to see why they have airway obstruction and any reversible causes addressed first. The patient may still need CPAP, but at least the chances of success are improved by reducing the severity of obstruction to start with.

Dental options

A significantly overlooked area of management in the process of sorting out upper airway obstruction is what a trained dentist can offer. They can offer minimally invasive options to improve the airway. This may mean the fitting of a special mouth guard, or using a device that mechanically pushes the jaw slowly outwards, to increase the dimensions of the jaws. I will go and explain each of these in a bit more detail, but as I am not a dentist, this is something that they can advise you about more so than any medically trained doctor can.

- Splints

Sometimes the simple use of an oral appliance that moves and holds the lower jaw slightly forwards makes enough of a difference to a patient's compromised airway that this is more than adequate management. This management option is really only suited for adults, but there are some trials going on exploring their use in children.

Whilst cheap versions can be bought over the internet, that is not such a great idea, as poorly fitting appliances can cause problems with the jaw joint. The integrity of these splints needs to be checked regularly, to make sure they are still doing the job they were designed for. One of the important things about these splints is that it is important for the nose to be nice and clear to breathe through. For this reason, many dental professionals that fit these appliances make sure patients see an ENT specialist first.

- Expansion

An expander is an orthodontic device that can be left inside the mouth for a couple of months and works by turning a small lever built within the device. By turning this lever, the mechanical arms of the device are leveraged in an outwards direction. This transmits a pressure force on to the jaw, and stretches it out. Apart from making the jaw wider, there is also some research that suggests it can make the space within the nose greater. This comes about because the nose sits on top of the upper jaw, and when the upper jaw moves out, the base of the nose does likewise. There is also some research suggesting that this technique can help to straighten a crooked nasal septum, which of course is a great added bonus for those with this contributing to their airway compromise.

Section 6. Outcomes of treatment of airway obstruction

There is very good evidence that managing upper airway obstruction in adults has a favourable outcome for adults. What I want to focus on here is whether getting in early with children makes a difference for the rest of their lives. In that regard I am going to focus on the more important aspects as follows:

- Brain function, with reference to behaviour, concentration, and school performance
- Heart, with reference to heart function and development
- Blood pressure, with reference to subtle vascular abnormalities
- Facial bones, with reference to their subsequent development

Whilst this book has made reference to the very many changes that come about in children with upper airway obstruction, the long and the short of it is that many things improve and return to normal. The reason for selecting these 4 specific areas is that they are by far the most important topics to focus on.

Brain function, with reference to behaviour, concentration, and school performance

The brain is an incredible thing. It is so complex, we can not understand it. However, we can investigate it and test it. Ultimately though, what we want to see is changes for the better. We want to see children do better at school, we want to see children behaving better, and we want to see children relate better with each other.

When parents become aware that the behavioural and learning problems their children are encountering may in some way relate to trouble with their breathing at night, most become very motivated to do whatever they can to get things sorted. But some ask "Can it wait for a few months?", "Is it urgent?", or even "At what age is it too late to see improvements?". These are really good questions. Hopefully the following serves as a reasonable attempt at answering them.

So the best place to start is to consider the question as to how long does upper airway obstruction have to be present to cause a problem. We do have some research that helps give us a guide on this. A research team monitored over 11,000 children for the first 7 years of their life. Their focus was on the presence of sleep disordered breathing in children through these early years, and the natural history of airway obstruction and subsequent outcomes in terms of concentration, behaviour, emotions, and inter-personal skills. To say the least, the results were quite enlightening.

First up, they found that any child who had sleep disordered breathing evident for at least 6 months at any age, whether it persisted or got better was way more likely by the age of 7 to demonstrate some form of behavioural or emotional problem. Furthermore, they found that the younger this happened, even if it got better quickly, it was still likely to leave a child with behavioural or emotional problems down the track. So the take home message from this research is that is only needs to be 6 months to do damage (it could be even less than this, but they were only assessing the children roughly every 6 months). The other important thing is that the earlier it occurs, the more vulnerable the children are to suffering consequences. The last aspect is that even though the upper airway obstruction may have a natural history of sorting itself out, the damage it does can otherwise potentially be permanent, so letting things be is not a great idea.

So that is a study where no interventions were carried out. The next logical step is to look at studies where children did have some form of intervention and see what changes came about. In this regard, there are lots of these studies, and the prime focus for most of them has been on school performance. But the first question to ask, of course is does having sleep disordered breathing actually affect school performance that much? The answer to this is overwhelmingly yes. Furthermore, we now know that the worse the obstruction is, the worse their performance at school is. Here is some perspective- children probably breathe about 15 times in a minute, which works out to 900 times in an hour. Studies have shown that children only need to have trouble breathing 6 times out of those 900 to run in to some serious problems.

Now to fixing things. The simple answer is yes, the studies show that children do improve at school when their airway obstruction if fixed. But what it also shows is that there is variability in just how much better things improve by. Also, as the children become older at the time point of fixing their problems, the less the improvements become. So the take home message there is that the sooner things are fixed the better.

They have also looked at children with a diagnosis of ADHD.
And long story short, it may be that up to 25% and maybe even 50% of children given this diagnosis actually have an underlying sleep problem, with sleep disordered breathing being the main type of sleep issue. Many studies have shown that children operated on for their airway issues that met the criteria for the diagnosis of ADHD improved so much after surgery that they no longer met the criteria for that diagnosis. In some countries in the world it is not permissible to commence medication for ADHD until a sleep assessment has been conducted.

Heart, with reference to heart function and development

The heart is one of those important things in the body that needs to work properly all of the time. There are several ways though that sleep problems can impact on heart function. Firstly, the heart needs to beat in a regular manner. This is called its rhythm. If its rhythm becomes irregular, then we call this an arrhythmia. In adults with OSA, they are at risk of a type of arrhythmia called atrial fibrillation. This is where one part of the heart beats faster than the rest. This impairs the pumping function of the rest of the heart. This results in patients feeling lethargic, light headed, and can be serious that it leads to having a stroke.

The rhythm of the heart is controlled internally by a series of electrical communications. We can measure this electrical activity using a machine called an ECG- you have more than likely seen this in action as it is an old favourite in TV shows- it is the machine that makes all the beeping noises and then all of a sudden stops to add some drama to the show. Anyway, in OSA, these circuits can misfire and we can measure this on an ECG.

Another way the heart can run into problems is that is has to pump against high pressure in the blood vessels. We covered this condition when we talked about hypertension, and there were two types of these- systemic and pulmonary. The heart can keep up with things to a degree, but when it starts to struggle we call this heart failure.

All of these things can happen in sleep disordered breathing with the last one in particular known to happen in children. In fact up to 20% of children with big adenoids have pulmonary hypertension and this puts them at risk of right sided heart failure. The good news is that to varying degrees, many of these heart problems become less of an issue once the airway obstruction is addressed. However, the best results are seen in children. So once again, the earlier the better when it comes to fixing things.

Blood vessel abnormalities other than high blood pressure

So far I have spoken broadly about problems with high blood pressure. Now I want to talk about the more subtle changes that can occur and of course how we can measure them.

The first is something called endothelial dysfunction. In simple terms, think about this- with one hand, grab a finger of the other, and with your thumb, push down on a finger nail or on the fingerprint tip of the finger on the other side, hold it for 10 seconds, and then let go. Notice how it blanches and then restores to its normal colour? This is a function of the blood vessels opening up to let blood back in rapidly. We can measure the time this takes. In people with sleep disordered breathing, this rate or refilling is slower. This is because the blood vessels are stiffer and do not stretch open as well as they should. In children this improves once the airway issues are sorted.

In sleep disordered breathing, we see an elevation in the bad cholesterol (called LDL), and a decrease in the good cholesterol (called HDL). This combination of events increases the chances of fatty deposits in the walls of the blood vessels, which leads to narrowing of the blood vessels over time. This is known as atherogenesis. Quite scarily we can see atherogenic changes in children. We also see this in adults that snore. It is not a good thing for your health when your blood vessels are getting blocked by fat.

Facial bones, with reference to their subsequent development

The debate over the development of facial bones and the potential influence of breathing patterns on this is a very emotive one. There are some dentists and orthodontists that feel that breathing has absolutely nothing to do with how the bones of the face and the jaws develop, and then there are those that are absolutely adamant that it does. The research on this is a real mixed bag. Some studies say it does, some studies say it doesn't.

So what can one believe?

The short answer is that you deal with an individual not studies. While the studies can guide your thoughts, if a child sitting in front of you is demonstrating a breathing problem, and they also have a problem with the way their jaw and face are developing, then you need to accept as a clinician that there are 2 problems in that child and that a team approach is necessary to work it all out. Arguing over whether it is related or not serves no purpose in a child that is suffering with more than one condition.

OK. That's me having a rant. What do I believe and what I do?

There are many studies showing children with orthodontic problems, when assessed by an ENT have a very high rate of airway problems. Furthermore, there are studies showing children with airway problems having a higher than expected rate of orthodontic problems. In other words, ignoring the potential cause and effect, we have children that when they have one problem are also likely to have the other. So on that basis, whether one causes the other is irrelevant. As the airway issues take precedence over crooked teeth, this is the first thing that should be assessed and managed. Some studies have even shown that by doing this, the orthodontic problems can improve by themselves. With the many dentists I work with, one part of the feedback that I get is that once I have helped a child to breathe better, the orthodontic treatment often goes better and works faster- I keep asking them to study this for me so we can publish the results, so maybe one day I will get my wish as we can add to the collective wisdom of this topic.

Section 7. Take home messages

This book has endeavoured to outline the many aspects of why the issue of upper airway obstruction can not be ignored. It also has intended to highlight the long-term consequences of a "wait and see" approach. In order to empower the parents of children, the following summary should serve as a worthwhile reference to allow for meaningful conversations with their health care provider.

A.   Snoring is a sign of upper airway obstruction

B.   Upper airway obstruction is a bad thing

C.   Mouth breathing is also an indication of upper airway obstruction

D.   A child that snores and/or mouth breathes 4 nights of the week or more should be referred to a Paediatric ENT specialist that has a special interest in upper airway obstruction

E.   There is an association between upper airway obstruction and:

   a) Behavioural problems

   b) Hearing problems

   c) Listening problems

   d) Memory problems

   e) School performance

   f) Bed wetting

   g) Blood noses, especially at night

h) ADHD

i) Jaw and orthodontic problems

j) Low energy levels

k) Low iron levels

l) Swallowing problems, and food avoidance

m) Sensitive gag reflex

n) High blood pressure

o) Heart problems

p) Visual problems

q) General body growth and development

r) Blood sugar regulation

s) High cholesterol

t) Low blood oxygen levels

u) Poor body posture

F. Surgery is the mainstay of treatment for children with upper airway obstruction, but additional therapy such as myofunctional training, medications, and dental intervention may also be important

G. There are many ways of performing surgery and it is important to understand how your specialist do their operations, and you should feel confident in asking about them which techniques they use so you are well informed

H. Tonsillitis is irrelevant when it comes to deciding upon surgical removal of the tonsils when there is airway obstruction

"The stupid lazy child who frequently suffers from headaches at school, breathes through his mouth instead of his nose, snores and is restless at night, and wakes up with a dry mouth in the morning, is well worthy of the solicitous attention of the school medical officer."

British Medical Journal

"On some causes of backwardness and stupidity in children"

Dr. William Hill in 1889

This was the first quote in this book, and is still the most important. Based on what has been outlined, let's go through this piece by piece.

Firstly, the days of having doctors at a school are behind us. Nonetheless, the principal recommendation was to see a doctor. This is back in the era before there were antibiotics and when "snake oil" merchants preying on the gullible public were aplenty. So what about the children that this quote made reference to?

Firstly, this book highlighted that children are not supposed to snore. If it is circumstantial such as having a cold, or being worn out from a big day, fair enough- but if it persists, then it is not normal.

Secondly, being a mouth breather is not a normal way to breathe. It affects the way the lungs can absorb oxygen into the blood. And children need every bit of oxygen they can get. Being a mouth breather also results in the mouth being dry come the morning.

Third, mouth breathing and snoring are symptoms of airway obstruction. Having restricted breathing sends emergency signals to the brain that something is wrong. These signals interfere with the brain's desire to have a rest and recharge its functional capacity for the next day. Constant signals to the brain interrupt the ability to have a rest, and results in a restless sleep.

Fourth, children getting poor quality sleep are not able to focus and concentrate on their education. There are easily distracted, and readily labelled as being "lazy".

Fifth, children who snore and mouth breathe may have issues with grinding their teeth, needing to arch their heads back to open their airway, and may have disrupted blood flow to their brains. All of these factors may contribute to having a headache.

So as you can see, they got it right over 125 years ago. In this modern era, to think that they were getting better sleep then, than we are now, is a sign that it is time to pause, look after our health, and make sure we are all getting a good night's sleep.

Further reading and help

By now you will have consumed a lot of information and it will take a while to digest it. Please read over it again and refresh your memory. For a professional assessment of your airway, appointments with Dr McIntosh can be made by looking up his clinic webpage entspecialists.com.au

Dr McIntosh is also a professional public speaker and you can contact him at david@entspecialists.com.au to discuss organising him to be present at your next function- he has spoken to a wide variety of audiences and can present on a wide range of informative topics.

There is a Facebook Page for this book- please like it, and share it and tag your friends to let them know how helpful the book was for you and that they should read it too. The page to search for is "Snored to Death".

Made in United States
Orlando, FL
26 July 2024

49569517R00104